W0228035

Hand Surgery Study Guide

Springer Science+Business Media, LLC

Steven F. Viegas

*Professor and Chief, Division of Hand Surgery, Department of
Orthopaedic Surgery; Professor of Anatomy and Neuroscience,
University of Texas Medical Branch, Galveston, Texas*

Hand Surgery
Study Guide

With Contributions by Patrick J. Kearney

Illustrations by Michael A. Cooley and Steven F. Viegas

With 107 Figures, 13 in Color

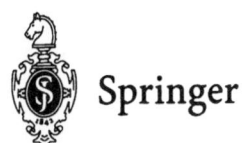 Springer

Steven F. Viegas, M.D.
Professor and Chief
Division of Hand Surgery
Department of Orthopaedic Surgery
and
Professor of Anatomy and Neuroscience
University of Texas Medical Branch
Galveston, TX 77555-0792
USA

Library of Congress Cataloging in Pubication Data
Viegas, Steven F.
    Hand surgery study guide / Steven F. Viegas.
        p.   cm.
    Includes bibliographical references and index.
    ISBN 978-0-387-94749-5   ISBN 978-1-4612-1910-1 (eBook)
    DOI 10.1007/978-1-4612-1910-1
    1. Hand – Surgery – Examinations, questions, etc. I. Title.
    [DNLM: 1. Hand Injuries – surgery – examination questions. WE 18.2
    V656h 1996]
    RD559.V54 1996
    617.5'75059'076 – dc20
    DNLM/DLC
    for Library of Congress   96-13742

Printed on acid-free paper.

© 1997 Springer Science+Business Media New York
Originally published by Springer-Verlag New York, Inc. in 1997

All rights reserved. This work may not be translated or copied in whole or in part without
the written permission of the publisher (Springer Science+Business Media, LLC), except for
brief excerpts in connection with reviews or scholarly analysis. Use in connection with any
form of information storage and retrieval, electronic adaptation, computer software, or by
similar or dissimilar methodology now known or hereafter developed is forbidden.
The use of general descriptive names, trade names, trademarks, etc., in this publication,
even if the former are not especially identified, is not to be taken as a sign that such names,
as understood by the Trade Marks and Merchandise Marks Act, may accordingly be used
freely by anyone.
While the advice and information in this book are believed to be true and accurate at the
date of going to press, neither the authors nor the editors nor the publisher can accept any
legal responsibility for any errors or omissions that may be made. The publisher makes no
warranty, express or implied, with respect to the material contained herein.

The material presented in the *Hand Surgery Study Guide* is for educational purposes. It is
hoped that this material will assist in the study and review of hand surgery. It is also
hoped that the reader will find the text helpful in preparation for the hand surgery
components of in-training, self-assessment, and recertification examinations. This material
is not suggested, however, to be used as the only text for review of hand surgery. The
methods, procedures, and treatments discussed are not necessarily suggested to be the
best or even those recommended by the authors.

Production managed by Allan Abrams and Terry Kornak; manufacturing supervised by
Joe Quatela.
Typeset by TechType, Inc., Ramsey, NJ

9 8 7 6 5 4 3 2 1

ISBN 978-0-387-94749-5

This book is dedicated to my family, the foundation from which, and upon which, all the rest of my life is built.

Preface

The field of hand surgery has grown tremendously in the past two decades. The knowledge base for this exciting and expanding field is voluminous and at times seemingly overwhelming for the student of hand surgery to begin to assimilate. The *Hand Surgery Study Guide* is recommended for students, residents, fellows, and practicing physicians as a quick reference to topics in hand surgery. This text is not written as a complete review of hand surgery. There are many fine hand surgery texts, journals, periodicals, and courses available to the student of hand surgery. Recommended readings are listed at the end of each chapter to assist the reader if more information is desired. The information presented in this text was selected based on the topics in hand surgery that have been covered over the past 20 years in the Orthopaedic In-Training Examination. Many of the topics have been revisited a number of times. Anyone who has taken on the effort of writing a question about a topic understands the difficulty of constructing a question that covers meaningful information, that is not controversial, and that is fair. This review text is a tribute to all of those individuals who made such an effort over the years.

Acknowledgments

To all those from whom I have learned and have been intellectually stimulated, including my students, residents, and colleagues, thank you. For those who will learn from this book I appreciate the time they will spend in its pages. I also wish to thank Dr. Mader, who reviewed the chapter on Hand Infections and Dr. Adesokan and Dr. Simmons, who helped in the selection of some of the photomicrographs for the Tumor chapter. Dr. Patrick J. Kearney, Division of Hand Surgery, Department of Orthopaedic Surgery, University of Texas Medical Branch, Galveston, contributed much of the material in Chapters 13 and 14. A thank you also to my ever-efficient, pleasant, and understanding secretary Mrs. Mary Moody, whose assistance in this effort, as in all the others, is much appreciated. Finally, a special thanks to Dr. E. Burke Evans for his continued support, encouragement, and mentorship.

Contents

1 Amputation and Replantation

In the past 30 years, replantation surgery has evolved from something to make medical headlines to something that is almost routine. There are now generally accepted indications and contraindications for replantation, as well as accepted techniques for replantation. With regard to appropriate candidates for replantation surgery, a traumatic amputation of the hand through the wrist in a young or middle-aged employed adult is generally considered an appropriate candidate for replantation. Single digits are generally not appropriate candidates, unless that digit is the thumb. The thumb is quite important functionally, and, in the event that replantation of the thumb cannot be accomplished and loss of the thumb is complete down to the level of the metacarpal head, appropriate treatment could include a microneurovascular free toe transfer. In a patient with clean, multiple-digit amputations, however, replantation of all the amputated parts would be considered an appropriate option. Multiple-level amputations of a digit or digits, crushing injuries, a warm ischemia time of over 24 hours, ring avulsion-type amputations, or amputations in psychotic individuals are generally cases that are considered contraindications for replantation surgery.

Ring avulsion injuries, in fact, are a well-accepted contraindication for replantation. Treatment should be amputation of the digit at the level of the injury, which can include skeletal shortening and primary wound closure. A seemingly less severe injury, such as a cut sustained from a ring traction-type of injury, should be recognized as a potentially more significant injury than merely a laceration. The vascularity of the digit should be examined, including Doppler examination if necessary and even a sympathetic block to see if circulation is intact or can be improved. If circulation is compromised, treatment should include microvascular repair.

Appropriate care of the amputated part is important in the success of replantation surgery. The amputated part should be wrapped in saline dressings, cooled in ice, and transported with the patient to the hospital.

The sequence of repair of structures in replantation of an amputated

1

digit is also important. Skeletal fixation should first be accomplished. In the case of a forearm or upper arm amputation, compression plating is the treatment of choice. Following skeletal stabilization, the tendons, arteries, veins, and, finally, skin closure should be the order of repair of the anatomic structures.

Single-digit amputation, other than the thumb, is a relative contraindication for replantation. The amputated stump should be revised or the hand reconstructed to optimize cosmesis and function. If the amputation is at the level of a joint with the articular cartilage intact, the articular cartilage should be removed and the wound closed primarily.

With regard to functional recovery, the best functional recovery is generally considered with replantations to be at the level of the DIP joint of the fingers or the IP joint of the thumb. Replantations through the base of the proximal phalanx can be expected to regain approximately half of PIP joint flexion and two-point discrimination of approximately 12 mm.

There are a number of complications that can occur in replantation surgery. Replantation of a hand amputated through the wrist can develop intrinsic muscle contractures, resulting in MP flexion and PIP extension contractures of all the fingers that would require an intrinsic muscle release. Stump pain and phantom limb pain can both be problems in patients with amputations. Surgical treatment of stump pain is generally more effective than the treatment of phantom limb pain. Postamputation limb pain in adults is most commonly associated with the level of the amputation and the presence of pain in that limb prior to amputation. Amputation of the distal portion of the finger or fingers can result in excessive pull on the lumbrical muscle by the proximal stump of the profundus tendon, which can result in the ability to flex the PIP joint when making a fist but inability to flex the PIP joint while maintaining the MP joint in extension or grasping a golf club or baseball bat. In major limb replantations at the level of the proximal one-third of the forearm or higher, it is important to perform adequate fasciotomies and muscle debridement since the most common cause of failure of major limb replantations is inadequate fasciotomy and muscle debridement. Adhesions of the flexor tendon(s) at the level of the amputation stump can also result in complications and limited function.

Recommended Reading

Glickman, L., and S. Mackinnon. 1990. Sensory recovery following digital replantation. Microsurgery 11:236.

Goldner, R. D., M. P. Howson, J. A. Nunley, et al. 1990. One hundred eleven thumb amputations: Replantation versus revision. Microsurgery 11: 243.

Urbaniak, J. R. 1993. Replantation. In: Operative hand surgery, ed. D. P. Green,

1085. New York: Churchill Livingstone.

Urbaniak, J. R., J. P. Evans, and D. S. Bright. 1981. Microvascular management of ring avulsion injuries. J. Hand Surg. 6:25.

Urbaniak, J. R., J. H. Roth, J. A. Nunley, R. D. Goldner, and L. A. Koman. 1985. The results of replantation after amputation of a single finger. J. Bone Joint Surg. 67A:611.

Questions

A. A 24-year-old carpenter amputates his left small finger at the middle of the middle phalanx. He is treated by primary closure of the amputation. His grip strength is still diminished 1 year later. He complains also of aching and cramping in the palm. The amputation stump has healed nicely, and the little finger has normal active motion. Active flexion of the distal interphalangeal joints of the long and ring fingers is normal when the proximal interphalangeal joints are held in extension; when these joints are not restricted, however, active flexion of the distal interphalangeal joints is limited and weak. The patient's condition is most likely due to:

1. Sublimis tendon adhesion in the palm
2. Profundus tendon adhesion at the amputation stump
3. Profundus tendon adhesion in the ring and long fingers
4. Lumbrical-plus fingers
5. Intrinsic muscle contracture

B. A 30-year-old man amputates the distal phalanx of his middle finger. Six months later, he complains of continued stiffness of his PIP joint. On examination, active PIP joint flexion with the MP joint held in extension is only 20°. However, when the MP joint is flexed, active PIP flexion is 90°. Which of the following treatments is most likely to correct this condition?

1. Release of the PIP joint collateral ligaments
2. Z-lengthening of the extensor tendon central slip
3. Release of the dorsal capsule and z-lengthening of the central extensor slip
4. Release and dorsal relocation of the lateral band's central extensor slip
5. Division of the lumbrical tendon

C. A 19-year-old woman sustains a ring avulsion injury with complete degloving of her right ring finger. Both neurovascular bundles are avulsed with the degloved skin. The skeleton and tendons are intact, and there are full active digital flexion and extension. Treatment should include:

1. Replantation of the degloved skin
2. Covering the digit with a pedicle flap

3. Covering the digit with a neurovascular island flap
4. Covering the digit with a split-thickness skin graft
5. Amputation of the finger and primary closure of the wound

D. In a middle-aged working man, which of the following would be the most appropriate for replantation?

1. Amputation of the ring finger through the proximal phalanx
2. Amputation of the index finger through the proximal phalanx
3. Amputation of the thumb through the nailbed
4. Amputation of the hand through the wrist
5. Amputation of the arm through the midhumerus

E. A 35-year-old, healthy truck driver presents to the Emergency Room 2 hours after having caught his wedding ring on his truck when jumping down to the ground. There is a circumferential laceration around his ring finger with partial extensor tendon injury. Flexor tendon function is intact. There is no fracture of the proximal phalanx. The left ring finger circulation is poor and the finger is pale distal to the laceration. The most appropriate treatment is:

1. Amputation and primary closure
2. Microvascular repair
3. Delayed tendon repair and wound closure
4. Cross finger flap
5. Island pedicle flap

2 Extensor Tendon Injuries

The extensor mechanism can be injured anywhere from the DIP joint to the proximal forearm. Disruption of the extensor mechanism at the level of the DIP joint of the finger, with or without a fracture fragment from the distal phalanx, can result in a characteristic flexion deformity called a "mallet finger." Hyperextension of the PIP joint may also be observed, due to an imbalance between flexor and extensor forces at the PIP joint (Fig. 2–1). Treatment of closed, acute mallet finger deformities is generally successful with a dorsal or volar splint which continually maintains the DIP joint in neutral or slight extension for a minimum of 6 weeks. Although in the past, operative treatment has been recommended for mallet finger injuries with fracture fragments involving more than one-third of the articular surface or volar subluxation of the distal phalanx, some now advocate that even these types of mallet finger injuries can be treated with splinting.

Disruption of the extensor mechanism at the level of the PIP joint where the central slip of the extensor tendon is disrupted and the lateral bands migrate in a volar direction will result in a so-called boutonniere deformity. This will result in loss of extension at the PIP joint and a compensatory hyperextension and possible limitation of flexion at the DIP joint (Fig. 2–2). This type of disruption of the extensor mechanism can result from a dorsal laceration over the PIP joint, blunt trauma to the dorsal area of the PIP joint causing disruption of the central slip, rupture or attenuation of the central slip due to PIP joint synovitis, and a volar dislocation of the PIP joint with resulting rupture of the central slip of the extensor mechanism (Fig. 2–3).

Treatment of a boutonniere deformity attempts to restore normal tendon length and balance by splinting the PIP joint in full extension, thereby approximating the ruptured, separated ends of the central slip and allowing active flexion of the DIP joint, which will move the lateral bands distally and dorsally. If successful, this will allow healing and contracture of the disrupted central slip to its anatomic length and mobilization of the lateral bands to their normal position, which is dorsal

A

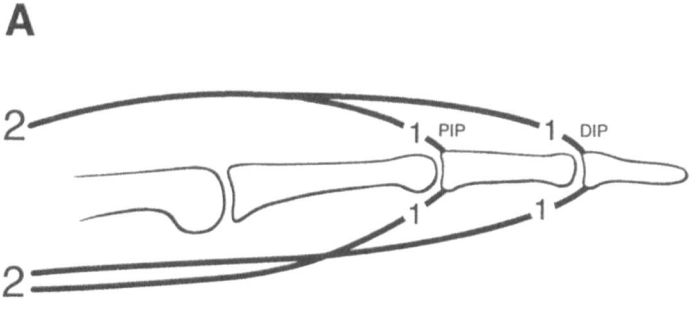

B

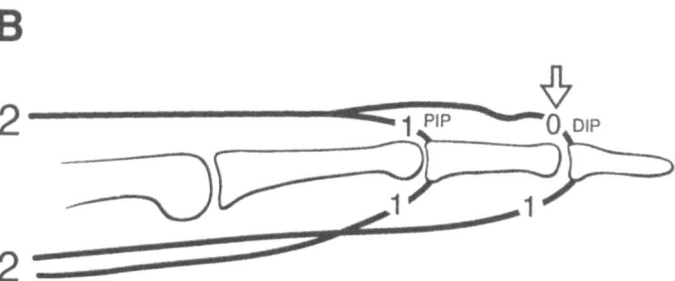

Fig. 2-1. (A) A simplified diagrammatic representation of the balance between extensor and flexor tendon insertions shows equal balance at the DIP and PIP joints. (B) Disruption of the extensor tendon at the DIP joint level.

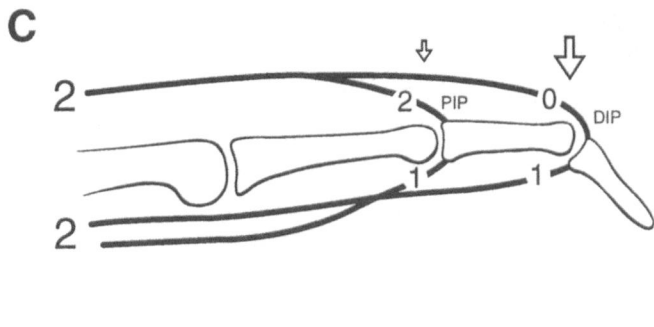

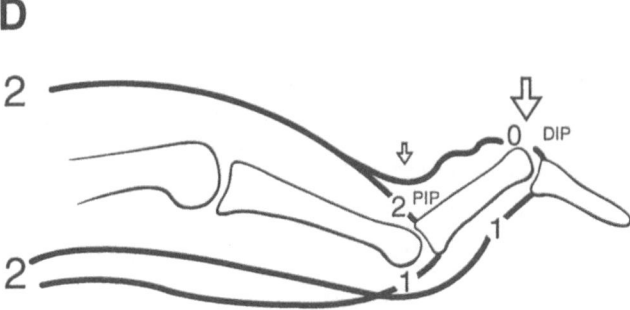

Fig. 2-1. (cont'd) (C) This results in an imbalance, and unopposed flexion at the DIP joint would result in a "mallet finger" deformity. (D) Subsequent imbalance at the PIP joint will result in hyperextension at the PIP joint, causing the so-called swan neck deformity.

A

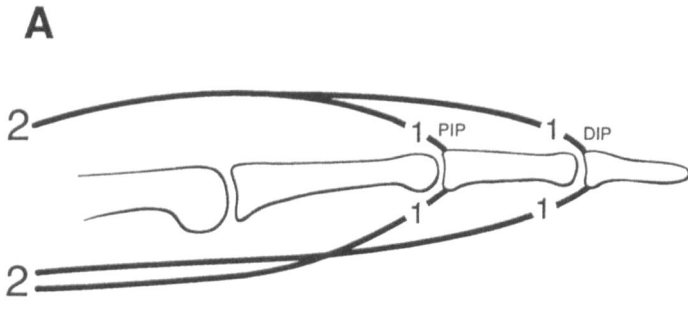

B

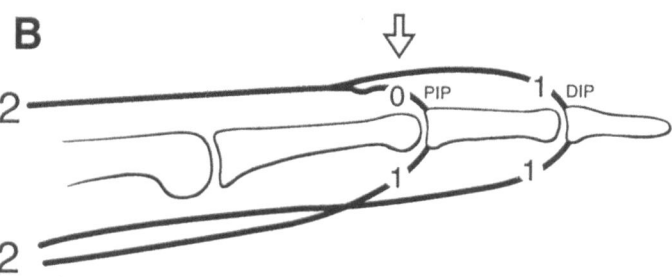

Fig. 2-2. (A) Using the same simplified diagrammatic representation of the balance between flexor and extensor tendons, (B) this time with a disruption of the extensor tendon at the PIP joint.

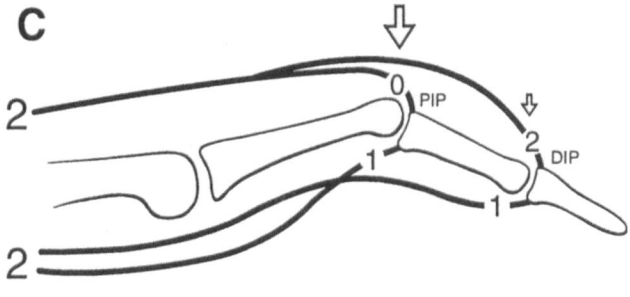

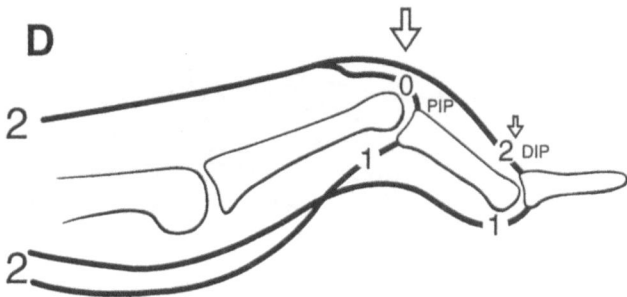

Fig. 2-2. (cont'd) (C) This results in unopposed flexion at the PIP joint (D) with resulting imbalance at the DIP joint causing hyperextension there. This results in the so-called boutonniere deformity.

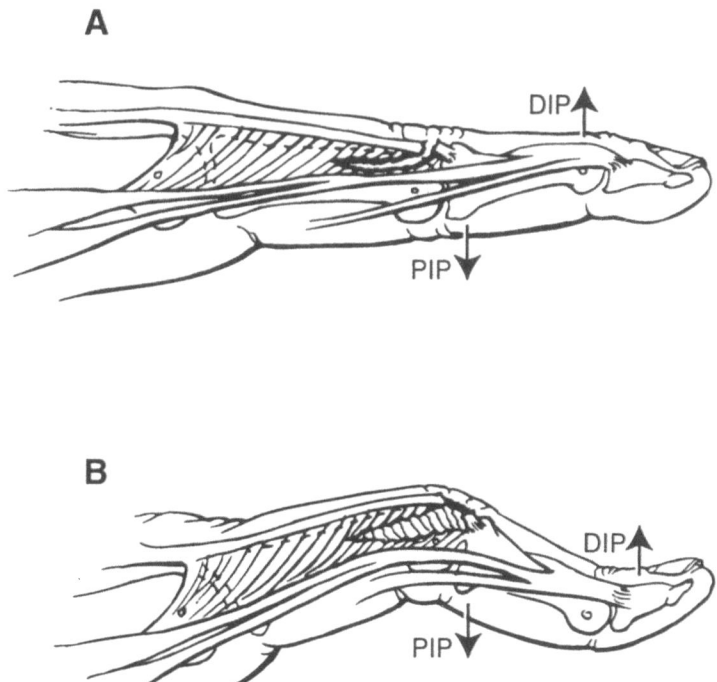

Fig. 2-3. A more accurate anatomic diagram of a boutonniere deformity shows (A) the tear through the central extensor slip and the extensor hood, which allows the lateral bands to sublux from their normal position, which is dorsal to the flexion axis at the PIP joint; (B) to a palmar position which not only fails to extend the PIP joint but, in fact, causes a greater flexion force at the PIP joint and hyperextension force at the DIP joint.

to the axis of rotation of the PIP joint. Dynamic extension splinting of the PIP joint, even in chronic and fixed deformities, is often useful. If this treatment fails or there is a bone fragment that has significantly migrated in a proximal direction and is lying over the PIP joint, these are situations in which surgical repair of the central slip and mobilization of the lateral bands to a more anatomic dorsal location would be appropriate.

The extensor pollicis longus tendon lies in the third of the six dorsal compartments (Fig. 2–4). Although not common, rupture of the extensor pollicis longus tendon following a distal radius fracture, even one that is nondisplaced, can occur. Physical examination may reveal lack of IP joint extension of the thumb and inability to lift the thumb off a tabletop when the hand and digits are placed palm down on the table. Also, tenderness to palpation may be present along the course of the extensor pollicis longus tendon. Rupture of the extensor pollicis longus tendon can be managed by transfer of the extensor indicis proprius tendon to the extensor pollicis longus distal tendon stump.

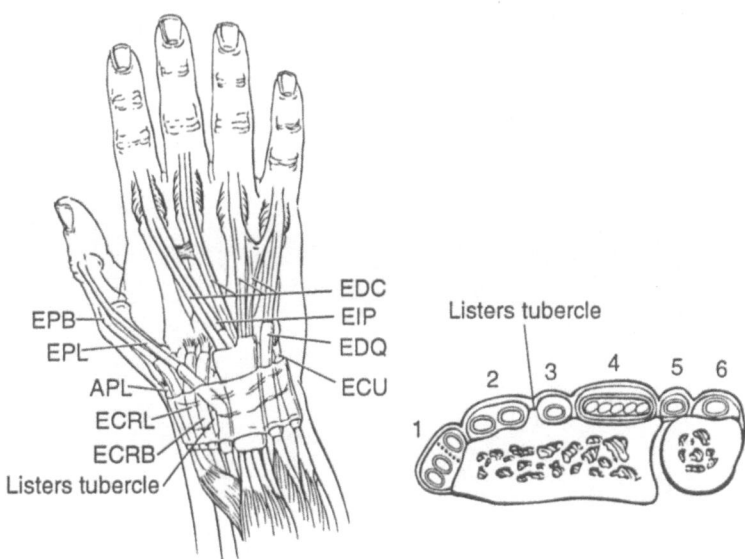

Fig. 2–4. Two illustrations, a dorsal view and a cross section, showing the anatomy of the extensor tendons and the extensor compartments. Extensor compartment 1 can have a septation (dotted line) within it, which forms a separate subcompartment for the extensor pollicis brevis tendon. (APL, abductor pollicis longus; EPB, extensor pollicis brevis; ECRB, extensor carpi radialis brevis; ECRL, extensor carpi radialis longus; EPL, extensor pollicis longus; EIP, extensor indicis proprious; EDC, extensor digitorum communis; EDQ, extensor digiti quinti; ECU, extensor carpi ulnaris.)

Patients with rheumatoid arthritis can develop dorsal extensor tenosynovitis and synovitis of the distal radioulnar joint. This may result in rupture most commonly at the distal border of the extensor retinaculum at the level of the distal radioulnar joint. The degenerative distal ulna can erode through the distal radioulnar joint capsule and, eventually, the extensor tendons (Fig. 2-5). It is important to be able to differentiate extensor tendon rupture from posterior interosseous nerve palsy, extensor mechanism subluxation, and MP joint dislocation. One of the means to examine and attempt to differentiate extensor tendon rupture from these other differential diagnoses is to determine if the fingers extend at the MP joint and IP joints when the wrist is passively flexed. This is called the "tenodesis effect" and should be present if the extensor tendons have not ruptured. Treatment of extensor tendon ruptures depends on how many of the tendons have been ruptured and whether direct repair of the tendons can be obtained, or instead tendon side-to-side transfers, should be performed, or, alternatively, the ruptures should be treated with tendon transfer or grafting.

Lacerations, fractures, or crush injuries can result in extensor tendon adhesions which, depending on the level of extensor tendon adhesions, will be evident by a discrepancy between active and passive range of motion.

A carpal-metacarpal boss may be the etiologic factor in a tendinitis of the third extensor digiti communis.

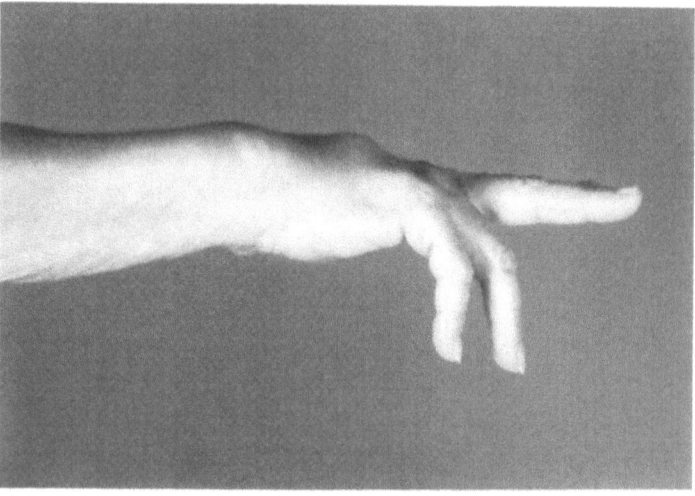

a

Fig. 2-5. (a) A clinical photo of a 57-year-old woman who is attempting to extend all the digits of her hand. It is noted that she is unable to extend the ring and little fingers, and there is an abnormal swelling over the dorsal aspect of the hand and wrist.

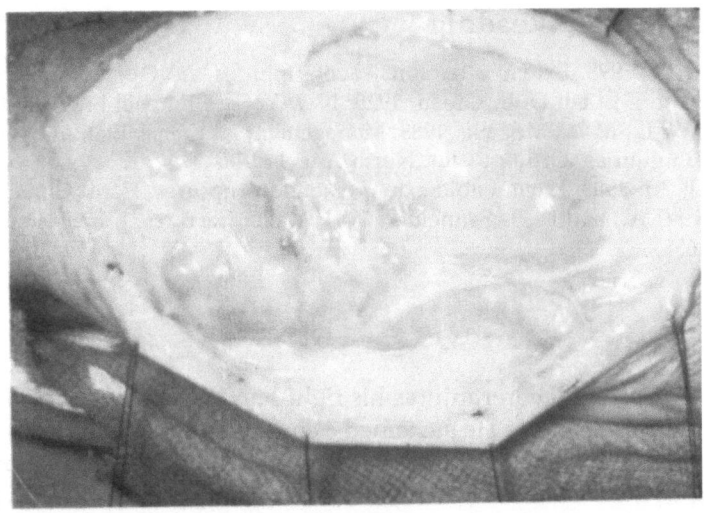

b

Fig. 2-5. (b) A dorsal incision exposing the attenuated extensor retinaculum.

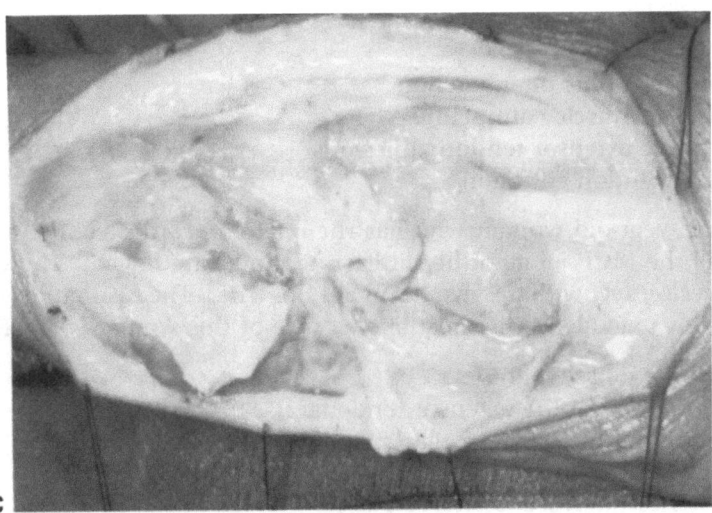

c

Fig. 2-5. (c) The incised and reflected extensor retinaculum with the ruptured ends of the extensor digitorum communis tendon to the ring and little fingers and the ruptured tendon of the extensor digiti minimi tendon.

Recommended Reading

Doyle, J. R. 1993. Extensor tendons—acute injuries. *In:* Operative Hand Surgery, 3rd Ed., ed. D. P. Green, 1925. New York: Churchill Livingstone.

Lovett, W. L., M. A. McCalla. 1983. Management and rehabilitation of extensor tendon injuries. Orthop. Clin. North Am. 14:811.

Leslie, B. M. 1989. Rheumatoid extensor tendon ruptures. Hand Clin. 5:191.

Wehbe, M. A., and L. H. Schneider. 1984. Mallet fractures. J. Bone Joint Surg. 66A:658.

Questions

A. A 27-year-old laborer injures his right hand when an I-beam temporarily pinned his hand. He sustained a comminuted, closed right second metacarpal fracture. The fracture healed with closed reduction and casting of the fracture. The man continued complaining of index finger stiffness and weakness of grip even 6 months after the fracture united. The patient now has PIP joint flexion with the MCP joint in 0° of extension, but only 25° of PIP joint flexion when the MCP joint is flexed to 90°. The MCP joint flexes to 40° when the PIP joint is also flexed, and 90° when the PIP joint is held in 0° of extension. The most likely diagnosis is:

1. Quadrigia effect
2. Lumbrical plus phenomenon
3. Intrinsic muscle contractures
4. Extrinsic extensor tendon adhesions
5. Flexor tendon adhesion

B. A 48-year-old woman who has rheumatoid arthritis cannot actively extend the MCP joints of her little, ring, and long fingers. There is no tenodesis effect with passive flexion of the wrist. The MCP joints can be passively extended. The most likely cause of this woman's problem is:

1. Intrinsic muscle tightness
2. Subluxation of the extensor tendons
3. Rupture of the extensor tendons
4. MCP joint dislocation
5. Posterior interosseous nerve palsy

C. A 39-year-old woman falls on her right wrist and sustains a transverse, minimally displaced fracture of the distal radius metaphysis. Three months later, she complains of dorsal wrist pain and decreased interphalangeal thumb extension. She has normal passive thumb and wrist motion. Active thumb interphalangeal motion is 30° to 60°. Radiographs show the healed fracture, without any other abnormalities. Treatment should consist of:

1. Exploration and decompression of the posterior interosseous nerve
2. Interphalangeal joint extension splinting
3. Third dorsal wrist compartment tenosynovectomy
4. Thumb MCP joint fusion and extensor pollicis brevis transfer to the extensor pollicis longus
5. Extensor indicis proprius to the extensor pollicis longus

D. An 20-year-old man "jams" his ring finger while playing volleyball. He develops diffuse proximal interphalangeal joint swelling and tenderness over the dorsal aspect of the PIP joint and a 30° flexion deformity at the joint. Passive motion of the PIP joint is normal. Active PIP joint motion is from 30° to 90°. When the PIP joint is positioned passively in 0° of extension, the young man is able to maintain this position actively. When the PIP joint is positioned passively in 90° of flexion, the young man is unable to actively extend the joint. X-rays are unremarkable. Treatment management should include:

1. Exploration and surgical repair of the central slip and the lateral bands
2. A PIP joint extension block splint which blocks extension beyond 30°
3. A dynamic PIP joint extension splint, which allows active PIP joint flexion
4. A static PIP joint extension splint, which allows active DIP joint flexion
5. A static PIP joint 30° flexion splint, which allows active DIP joint flexion

3 Flexor Tendon Injuries

Each of the fingers has a flexor digitorum sublimis tendon and a flexor digitorum profundus tendon. The flexor digitorum profundus tendons have a common muscle belly and are interconnected at the musculotendinous junction, thereby restricting independent profundus excursion, resulting in combined motion of all four profundus tendons with the so-called quadrigia effect. The blood supply to the flexor tendons is obtained from the dorsal side of the tendons through the vinculae. Core sutures used in the repair of lacerated tendons should be placed in the palmar half of the tendon to help preserve the dorsal blood supply. Although at one time it was recommended not to repair both tendons and, in fact, occasionally to excise the stump of the sublimis, it is now generally accepted that the appropriate treatment should be repair of both tendons. This has the advantage of maintaining the vincula system and, therefore, the blood supply to the tendons (Fig. 3-1).

The level at which the tendons will be lacerated in relation to the skin laceration will vary depending on the posture of the hand during the time of the injury. When the hand is flexed, such as when grasping a knife, the distal flexor tendon stumps will generally be found distal to the skin laceration; because of the difference in excursion of the profundus tendon, compared to the sublimis, the cut ends of the profundus and sublimis will be at different levels. The recommended treatment for uncontaminated lacerations of the digits is primary or delayed primary repair of all of the digital nerves and flexor tendons.

The tensile strengths of different tendon suture techniques has found that the Bunnell and Kessler sutures were the strongest initially, but the Kessler suture was strongest on the fifth day. From the 10th day on, there was no significant difference, although the Bunnell suture technique is felt to have a constricting effect on the tendon and its blood supply which the Kessler technique would not have. The original Kessler technique had suture knots that were left exposed; therefore, the modified Kessler-Tajima suture technique buries the knots within the repair site. More recently, a number of new suturing techniques

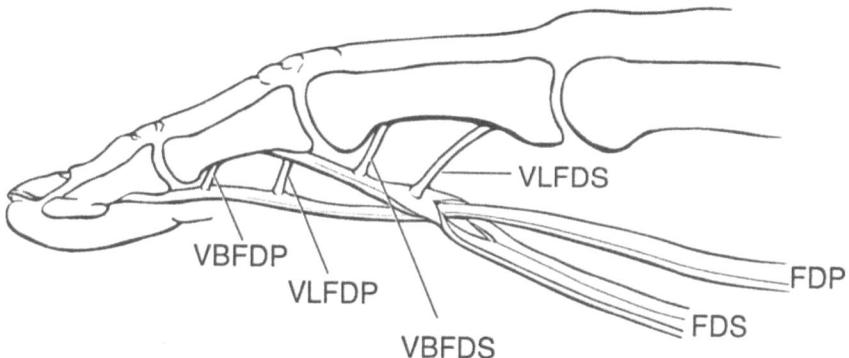

Fig. 3-1. The vincula longus and brevis to the flexor digitorum sublimis tendons and the vincula longus and brevis to the flexor digitorum profundus tendons. (VLFDS, vincula longus to the flexor digitorum sublimis; VBFDS, vincula brevis to the flexor digitorum sublimis; VLFDP, vincula longus to the flexor digitorum profundis; VBFDP, vincula brevis to the flexor digitorum profundis.)

have been developed that reportedly are stronger with less tendency for tendon gaping at the repair site.

Flexor tendon repair is considered weakest at 7 to 10 days. The A2 and A4 pulleys are considered the most important of the pulley system, and 80% of finger flexion can still be maintained if these two pulleys are intact. If the entire pulley system is disrupted, the A2 and A4 pulleys, at least, would need to be reconstructed. If the pulley system is not adequately preserved or reconstructed, "bow-stringing" of the flexor tendons can be observed and loss of full flexion can result. The A1 pulley is the site of tenderness and catching or locking in the trigger finger or trigger thumb. The radial digital nerve of the thumb is at greater risk of injury during surgical release of the A1 pulley of the thumb for treatment of trigger thumb (Fig. 3-2).

Postoperative immobilization and rehabilitation for flexor tendon injuries should maintain the wrist initially in 30° of flexion with 70° of MCP joint flexion, and early supervised active digital extension with passive flexion through dynamic traction upon the fingers.

A number of problems or complications can result from flexor tendon repairs. A distal laceration of the flexor profundus can be treated with surgical advancement of up to 1 cm and reinsertion of the profundus tendon. However, if the profundus tendon is advanced too far distally, flexion contracture at the DIP and PIP joints can result and/or flexion can become limited in the adjacent digits, due to a secondary laxity in the profundus tendons to the adjacent fingers, due to the quadrigia effect. If the flexor tendon graft or a flexor tendon repair or advancement results in flexor tendon shortening, there can be a combined lack of active interphalangeal joint extension while individual joints may still

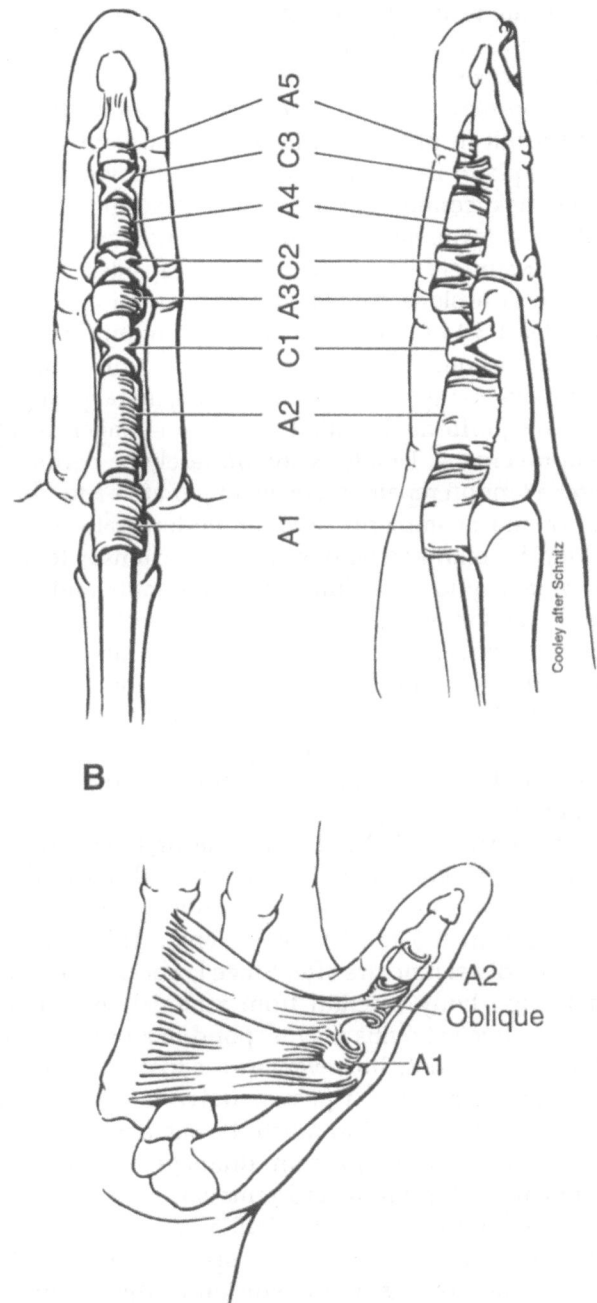

Fig. 3-2. (A) The pulley system of the fingers and (B) the pulley system of the thumb.

have full extension when the adjacent joints are held in full flexion. Alternatively, if the profundus is lacerated and retracts proximally or a flexor tendon graft is used for repair or reconstruction and its length is excessive, the increased excursion of the proximal stump of that grafted profundus tendon may result in excessive traction on the lumbrical to that digit and result in proximal interphalangeal joint extension when the patient attempts to flex that finger. This is known as "paradoxical" extension. The most common problem after flexor tendon grafting and repair is adhesion formation. Capsular scarring can also occur if the laceration and/or surgery is around the joint capsules.

Flexor tendon adhesions should be treated with aggressive physiotherapy for at least 3 to 6 months following tendon repair or grafting. Flexor tendon adhesions will typically result in a discrepancy between active and passive range of motion. It is generally suggested that tenolysis not be performed until therapy no longer results in any functional improvement. Tenolysis should rarely be performed prior to 3 months after a tendon repair and even longer after a tendon graft. The tendons that are most commonly used for tendon grafts are the palmaris longus tendon, the plantaris tendon, and toe extensor tendons.

Septic flexor tenosynovitis is important to identify and, if left untreated, can lead to tendon adhesions and even necrosis and rupture of the flexor tendons. Kanavel described four cardinal signs of septic flexor tenosynovitis: (1) pain on passive extension; (2) tenderness to palpation along the tendon sheath; (3) swelling along the tendon sheath; and (4) a flexed posturing of the finger. Appropriate treatment of septic flexor tenosynovitis should include incision, drainage, irrigation, and appropriate IV antibiotics.

In the postoperative period following the first stage of a two stage flexor tendon reconstruction in which a silastic rod is placed in the flexor tendon sheath, culture-negative postoperative synovitis of the sheath has been reported in 8% to 20% of patients. This may result from breakdown of the distal juncture after Stage I, buckling or binding of the implant, or foreign body reaction from material such as talc on the implant. This reactive synovitis may respond to a period of immobilization. The burden of proof, however, in a situation such as this is to demonstrate that there is not a postoperative infection. If infection is present, this should be treated in much the same way as a septic flexor tenosynovitis, which includes incision, drainage, irrigation, and appropriate IV antibiotics, plus silastic rod removal.

A common finger injury seen in football players is the so- called jersey finger in which there is a forceful and abrupt extension of the flexed PIP and DIP joints which results in an avulsion of the profundus tendon. Usually, this injury occurs in the ring finger. Several types of this injury have been classified.

Type I. The tendon retracts into the palm, rupturing the vincula with a resulting disruption of the blood supply to the profundus tendon. On physical examination, there is a tender mass in the palm. This tendon should be reinserted within 7 to 10 days before it becomes contracted.

Type II. The most common type, where the tendon retracts to the level of the PIP joint and the vincula at this level is intact. This type is best treated by early reinsertion of the tendon into the distal phalanx. However, in contrast to Type I injuries, the repair can be performed up to 3 months or more postinjury, due to the intact blood supply to the tendon.

Type III. There is a large, bony fragment avulsed with the profundus tendon which does not retract proximal to the A4 pulley because the avulsion fracture fragment cannot pass through the A4 pulley. Both vincula are usually intact. The bony fragment can be seen on lateral radiographs and may sometimes be palpated. Early reinsertion of the fragment with internal fixation is recommended in this type of lesion. A variant of this Type III injury has been described and is now called Type IIIA, in which there is a concomitant avulsion of the profundus tendon from the fracture fragment. Recommended treatment for this type of injury is internal fixation of the fracture fragment and then reinsertion of the avulsed profundus tendon. A late complication seen in the un-treated "jersey finger" can be a lumbrical plus finger in which the patient finds that the PIP joint begins to extend as the MCP joint reaches full flexion, due to excessive traction on the lumbrical muscle to that finger due to retraction of the proximal profundus tendon stump. This is another example of "paradoxical" extension.

Rupture of the flexor tendons can occur following distal radius fractures and as a result of carpal irregularities, wrist synovitis, or palmar carpal subluxation into the carpal tunnel. Rupture of the flexor pollicis longus from this type of pathology has been called the Manner-felt syndrome.

Recommended Reading

Leddy, J. P. 1993. Flexor tendon—acute injuries. *In:* Operative hand surgery, 3rd Ed., ed. D. P. Green, 1823. New York: Churchill Livingstone.

Schneider, L. H., and J. M. Hunter. 1993. Flexor tendons—late reconstruction. *In:* Operative hand surgery, 3rd Ed., ed. D. P. Green, 1853. New York: Churchill Livingstone.

Strickland, J. W. 1985. Flexor tendon repair. Hand Clin. 1:55.

Urbaniak, J. R., Cahill, J. D. Jr., and R. A. Mortinson. 1975. Tendon suturing methods: analysis of tensile strengths. *In:* The American Academy of Ortho-paedic Surgeons' Symposium on Tendon Surgery in the Hand, 70. St. Louis: C. V. Mosby.

Verdan, C. 1960. Syndrome of the quadrigia. Surg. Clin. North Am. 40:425.

Questions

A. An 18-year-old boy lacerates the flexor profundus of the long finger between the DIP and PIP flexor creases. He was treated by surgically advancing the profundus 1.5 cm and reinserting it into the distal phalanx. Three months later, the patient was unable to flex the index and ring fingers to the palm. The most likely cause of the patient's problem is:

1. Extensor tendon adhesions
2. Flexor tendon adhesions
3. Laxity of the profundus tendons to the index and ring fingers
4. Rupture of the repair
5. Tight lumbricals to the index and ring fingers

B. A 28-year-old laborer had his right hand pinned under an I-beam. He sustained displaced, closed, right index, middle, and ring finger proximal fractures. The fractures were reduced, closed, and immobilized with a splint in normal alignment. Three months later, the man complains of limited digital flexion and difficulty grasping small objects. He has normal active MCP motion, with active PIP joint motion from 0° to 45° and active DIP joint motion from 0° to 20°.

   Passive PIP joint motion is 0° to 90°, and passive DIP motion is 0° to 60°. The most likely cause of this impairment is:

1. Flexor tendon adhesions
2. Extensor tendon adhesions
3. Extensor tendon rupture
4. Flexor tendon rupture
5. PIP joint capsular scarring

C. A 26-year-old construction worker presents with a 3-day history of pain and swelling in his right index finger. He has some superficial abrasions on the palmar aspect of the finger. The index finger is swollen and held in slight flexion. He is tender over the palmar surface of the digit and has severe pain when the digit is passively extended. His temperature is 38°C and his WBC IS 11,500. The most likely diagnosis is:

1. Cellulitis
2. Septic arthritis, proximal interphalangeal joint
3. Septic arthritis, metacarpal phalangeal joint
4. Septic flexor tenosynovitis
5. Gout

D. An 18-year-old high school football player is seen 10 days after a game in which he injured the ring finger of his nondominant hand. He thinks that it occurred when he attempted to tackle another football player. The finger is mildly swollen, ecchymotic, and tender along the palmar surface. There is a tender mass in the palm. Radiographs reveal only soft tissue swelling. Figure 3-3 shows the appearance of the fingers

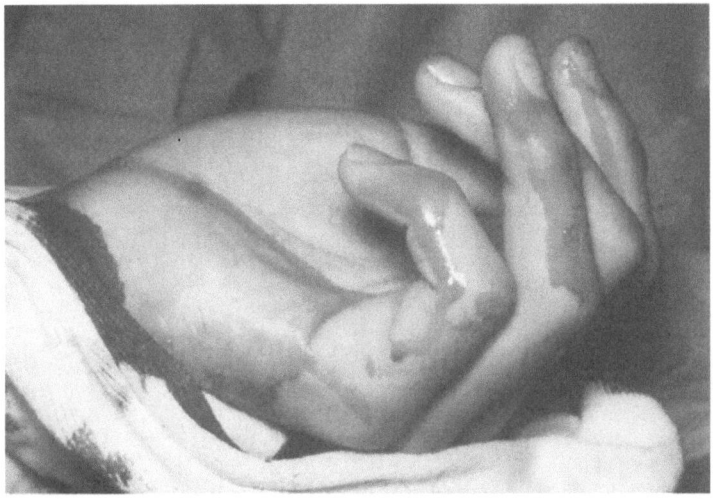

Fig. 3-3.

of the nondominant hand. Treatment should consist of:

1. Arteriography
2. Incision and drainage
3. Incisional biopsy of the mass
4. Tendon repair
5. Lumbrical reattachment

E. A 20-year-old man injured his right ring finger when he attempted to make a tackle by grabbing a player's shirt during a football game. He did not seek any medical care and had no initial treatment. Three months later, the patient cannot actively flex the DIP joint, though passive flexion is normal. When the patient attempts to flex the finger, the PIP joint begins to extend as the MCP joint approaches full flexion. The diagnosis most likely is:

1. An extension contracture of the proximal interphalangeal joint
2. Adhesion of the flexor digitorum profundus to the middle phalanx
3. A contracture of the fourth dorsal interosseous muscle
4. Lumbrical-plus finger
5. Quadrigia syndrome

4 Soft Tissue Coverage

Over the years, there have been a number of new techniques developed for soft tissue coverage of wounds of the hand. There is a smaller number of procedures that are generally accepted as reliable and have a high success rate. There are some that are particularly useful in certain areas of the hand. When there is soft tissue loss of up to 2.5 cm over the volar distal thumb tip, a volar advancement flap is often the procedure of choice (Fig. 4–1). When there is soft tissue loss over the volar aspect of the fingers, a cross finger flap is the procedure of choice (Fig. 4–2). A split-thickness skin graft, which includes the epidermis and partial thickness of the dermis, is used to cover the donor site resulting from the cross finger flap. When there is a sufficiently large soft tissue loss over the dorsum of the hand that cannot be addressed by primary closure, a radial volar forearm flap is one method for soft tissue coverage in that area (Fig. 4–3).

A longitudinal incision or scar oriented perpendicular to the flexor creases of the hand, particularly the digits, can result in a cosmetic and a functional impairment. A scar like this can be revised with a z-plasty to improve its appearance and lessen any functional impairment. A 60° angled z-plasty will result in a 75% increase in the length of the longitudinal scar (Fig. 4–4).

There are several concepts that are generally agreed upon with regard to certain soft tissue injuries. Ring avulsion injuries of the digits have sufficient soft tissue trauma that replantation, or, alternatively, soft tissue coverage of the stump is considered to be contraindicated. The accepted treatment of ring avulsion degloving injuries of the digits is skeletal shortening and primary closure. Amputations through the IP joints of the fingers are often best treated by surgical removal of the articular cartilage and primary closure of the wound. Most situations of soft tissue loss, including amputation of finger or thumb tips in toddlers, should be treated by local wound care. Generally, contaminated dirty wounds in the hand should be treated primarily with local wound care and delayed closure or soft tissue coverage.

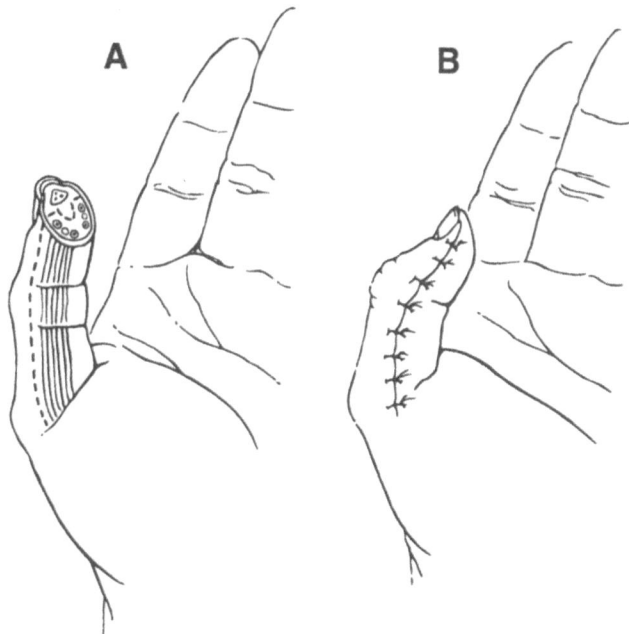

Fig. 4–1. (A) An illustration of a distal thumb tip amputation showing soft tissue loss and loss of the distalmost portion of the distal tuft of that thumb. (B) The volar advancement flap in which the volar flap is elevated surgically with the neurovascular bundles and advanced distal to cover the tip of the thumb.

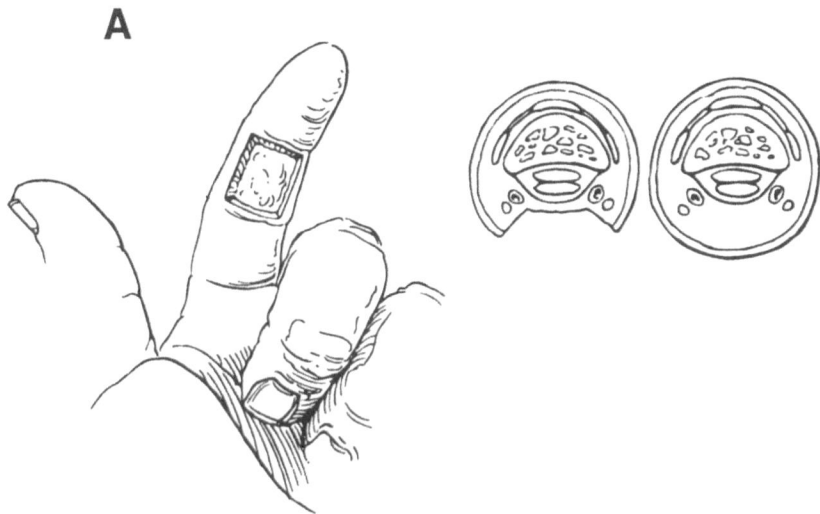

Fig. 4–2. (A) The overall appearance and cross-sectional schematic of a soft tissue loss over the volar aspect of an index finger.

B

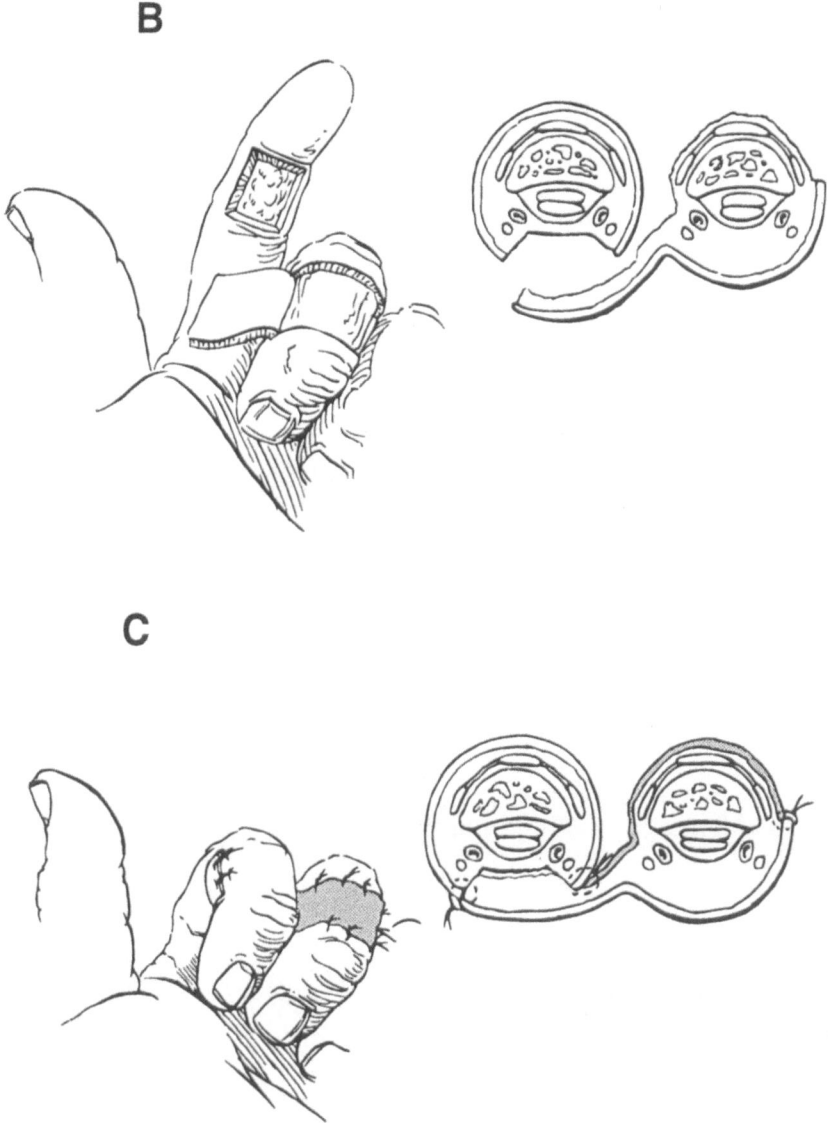

C

Fig. 4-2. (B) The elevation of a dorsal flap from the adjacent long finger. (C) Insertion of the flap to cover the soft tissue defect of the digit and a split-thickness skin graft (shaded area) used to cover the defect left from the use of the cross finger flap. The two digits are maintained like this for 2 to 3 weeks for adequate local blood supply to be established, at which point the fingers are divided surgically.

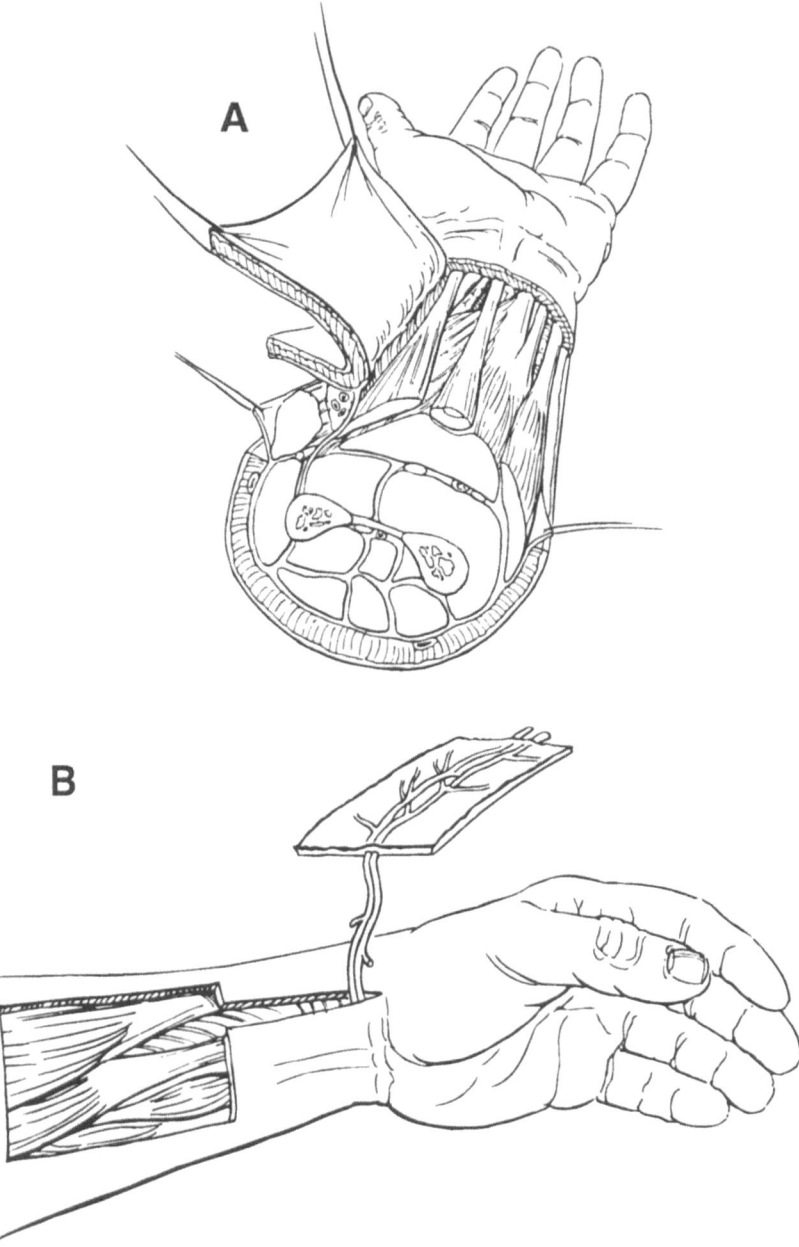

Fig. 4–3. (A) Dissection plane to establish a volar forearm flap based on a radial artery and the accompanying venous complex. (B) The radial forearm flap is mobilized on its distal radial artery pedicle.

C

D

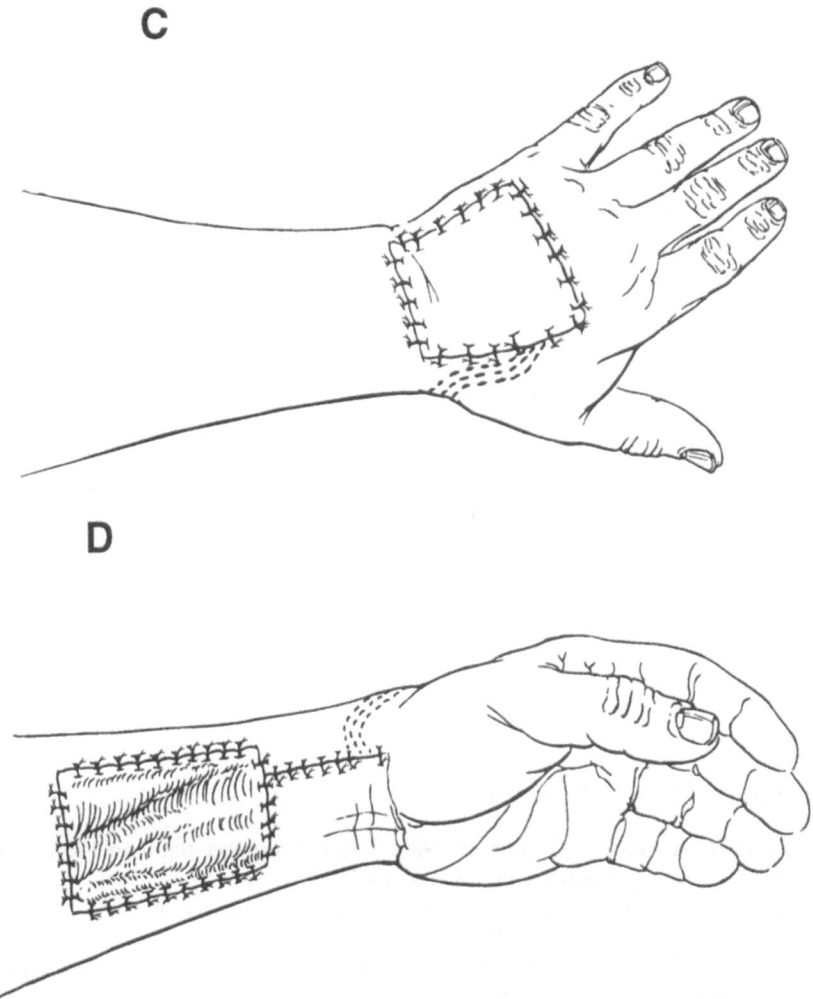

Fig. 4-3. (C) The pedicle and radial forearm flap is tunneled subcutaneously around the radial aspect of the wrist to deliver the radial forearm flap to cover a dorsal hand defect. (D) The soft tissue defect on the volar aspect of the forearm is covered with a split-thickness skin graft.

A   **B**

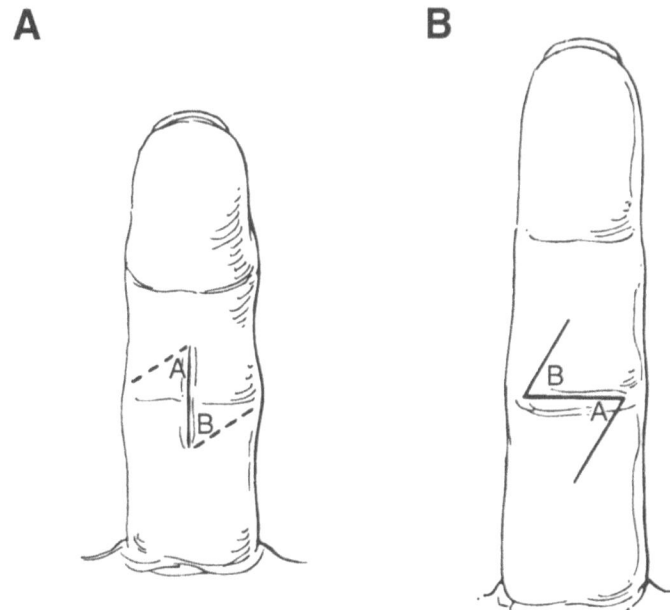

Fig. 4-4. (A) A scar contracture can be treated with (B) a simple 60° angled z-plasty, resulting in a 75% increase in the length of the original longitudinal scar.

Recommended Reading

Kappel, D. A., and J. G. Burech.1985. The cross-finger flap: an established reconstructive procedure. Hand Clin 1:677.

Lister, G. D. 1993. Skin flaps. *In:* Operative hand surgery, ed. D. P. Green, 2:1741. New York: Churchill Livingstone.

Moberg, E. 1964. Aspects of sensation in reconstructive surgery of the upper extremity. J. Bone Joint Surg. 46A:817.

Soutar, D.S. and N. S. B. Tanner. 1984. The radial forearm flap in the management of soft tissue injuries of the hand. Br. J. Plastic Surg. 37:18.

Questions

A. A 33-year-old, right-hand-dominant carpenter injures the tip of his right thumb in a table saw accident. Clinical examination reveals a 1.5 × 2.5 cm area of palmar skin and pulp loss with exposed bone. The nail is intact and there is full active IP joint flexion. The physician should recommend tetanus prophylaxis, parenteral antibiotics, wound debridement, and:

1. Local wound care, daily soaks, and dressing changes
2. A split-thickness skin graft
3. A full-thickness skin graft
4. A volar advancement flap
5. A cross finger flap from the little finger

B. A 20-year-old man injures the palmar surface of his right ring finger with a chain saw. The wound is irrigated and debrided of nonviable tissue which results in a 1.5 × 2 cm soft tissue defect. The A4 pulley, the flexor digitorum profundus, and the digital nerves are exposed. The wound should be covered with a:

1. Thenar flap
2. Cross finger flap
3. Lateral arm pedicle flap
4. Neurovascular island flap
5. Full-thickness skin graft

C. A 23-year-old man is involved in a motor vehicle accident and sustains a crush avulsion injury to his right hand. Following several debridements and plate fixation of multiple metacarpal fractures, the wound appears clean. However, there is a 4 × 5 cm soft tissue loss, including extensor tendon defects, with exposed plates on the dorsum of his hand. Culture results are negative. Treatment should now consist of:

1. Split-thickness skin grafting and extensor tendon grafting
2. Full-thickness skin grafting now and extensor tendon grafting as a second stage
3. Removal of plates and skeletal shortening with wound closure
4. A local rotation flap now, and extensor tendon reconstruction as a second stage
5. A radial volar forearm flap now, and extensor tendon reconstruction at a second stage

D. A 4-year-old boy amputates the tip of his right thumb. The nail bed is uninjured, but bone can be seen in the base of the wound. Management should consist of cleaning the wound and:

1. Local wound care A split thickness skin graft
2. A cross finger flap
3. A V-Y advancement flap
4. Shortening the distal phalanx and primary closure

5 Wrist Injuries

There are eight carpal bones and the radius and ulna which, together, form four separate joint spaces (Fig. 5-1). Normally, an arthrogram of the distal radioulnar joint will show dye contained within that space, unless there is a disruption of the triangular fibrocartilage complex, which would allow dye leakage into the proximal wrist joint (Fig. 5-2). An arthrogram of the midcarpal wrist joint would contain the dye within the midcarpal joint and between the scapholunate and lunotriquetral joints, unless there is disruption of the interosseous ligament so that the proximal carpal row would allow dye leakage into the proximal wrist joint. An arthrogram of the proximal wrist joint should be contained within that wrist joint, unless disruption of ligaments or the TFC allows dye leakage into the midcarpal and/or distal radioulnar joint. A fourth joint space, which is the pisotriquetral joint, can be seen regularly to communicate with the proximal wrist joint.

The recognition and understanding of carpal instabilities has increased tremendously over the past decade (Fig. 5-3). The most common type of carpal instability is a dorsal intercalated segment instability, a so-called DISI deformity (Fig. 5-4). Plane X-rays are helpful in determining carpal instabilities. A DISI deformity is most commonly caused by disruption of the scapholunate interosseous ligament, the radioscapholunate, and radioscaphocapitate ligaments. Plane X-rays would typically demonstrate an increased space between the scaphoid and lunate on an AP projection, particularly on a supinated, clenched fist view (Fig. 5-5); on a lateral view, the scapholunate angle would be greater than the normal 60° to 70° scapholunate angle (Fig. 5-6). Clinically, there can be dorsal tenderness over the scapholunate joint and a symptomatic clicking, as well as pain and a click when pressure is applied over the palmar aspect of the scaphoid tubercle as the wrist is deviated radially, which is the scaphoid stress test. Treatment of a scapholunate dissociation has been addressed in several ways. For a period of time, attempts at ligament reconstruction were done but subsequently were felt to be unpredictable. More recently, there was a

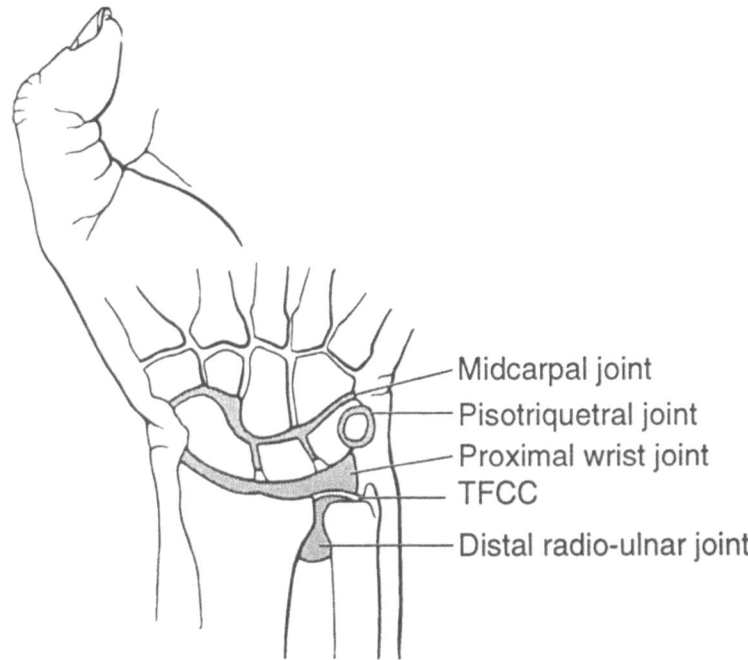

Fig. 5-1. An illustration of a section through an adult hand showing the four separate compartments that can be seen in wrist arthrography. These are the midcarpal joint, the proximal wrist joint, the distal radioulnar joint, and the pisotriquetral joint. The pisotriquetral joint can often communicate with the proximal wrist joint. (TFCC, triangular fibrocartilage complex.)

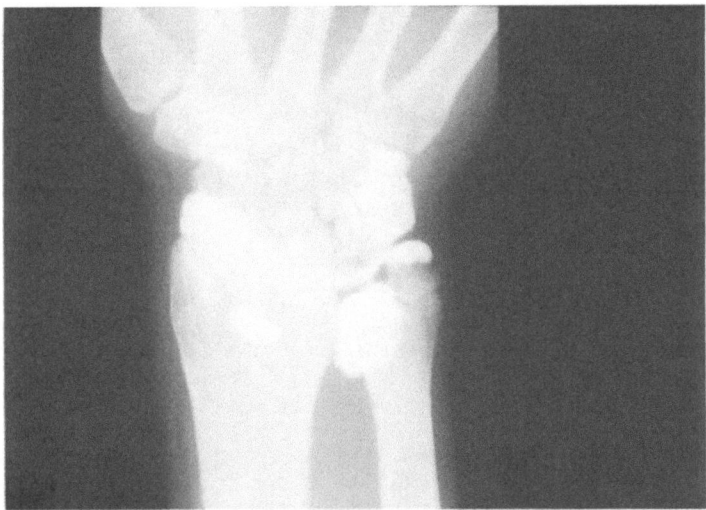

Fig. 5–2. An arthrogram demonstrating communication of the dye between the distal radioulnar joint and the proximal wrist joint, which results from a disruption in the triangular fibrocartilage complex.

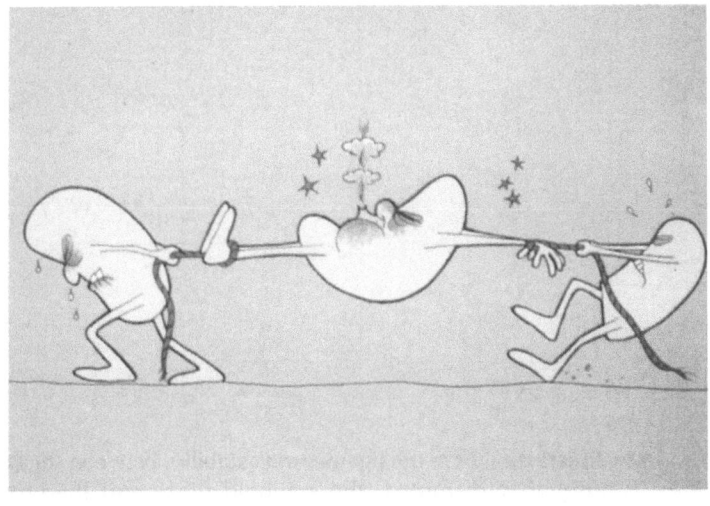

a

Fig. 5–3. The general understanding of the scaphoid, lunate, and triquetrum is that they are under constant and varying degrees of tension, with the tendency for the triquetrum to pull the lunate into extension and the scaphoid to pull the lunate into flexion. (a) Under normal conditions, the carpal bones of the proximal row are in balance.

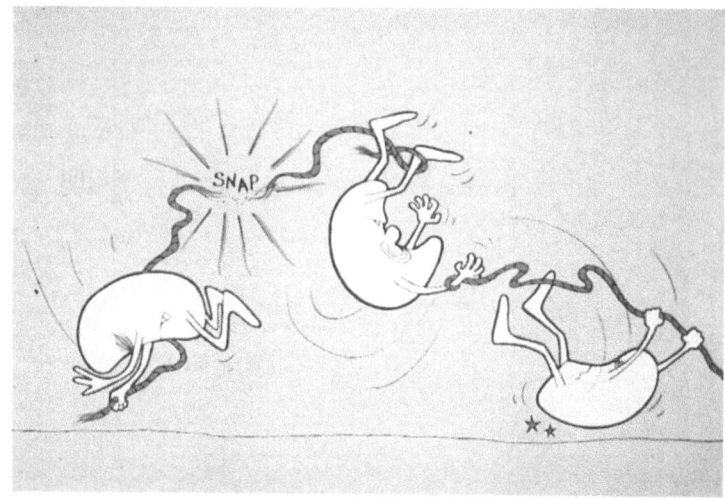

b

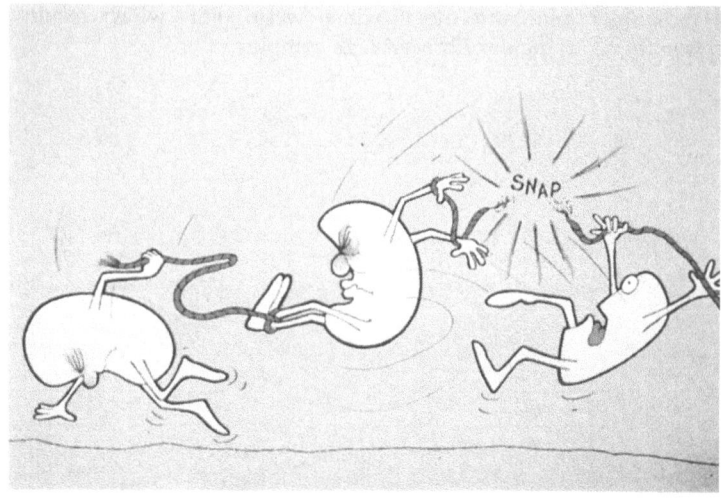

c

Fig. 5-3. (b) In situations where the ligamentous stability between the scaphoid and lunate is adequately disrupted, the scaphoid flexes and the lunate and triquetrum assume an extended posture. This is generally considered to result in a dorsal intercalated segment instability (DISI). (c) It has been generally believed that a similar disruption between the lunate and triquetrum will allow the triquetrum to assume a somewhat extended posture, while the lunate and scaphoid assume a flexed posture. The importance of the dorsal capsule and radiolunotriquetral ligament in preventing this type of instability has more recently been recognized in the pathomechanics of a volar intercalated segment instability (VISI).

B

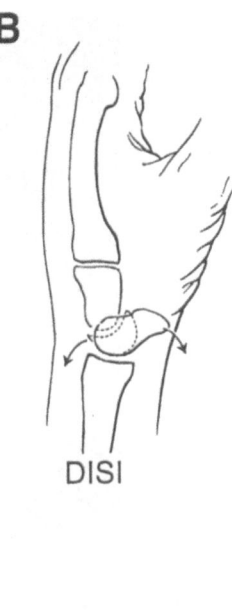

DISI

A

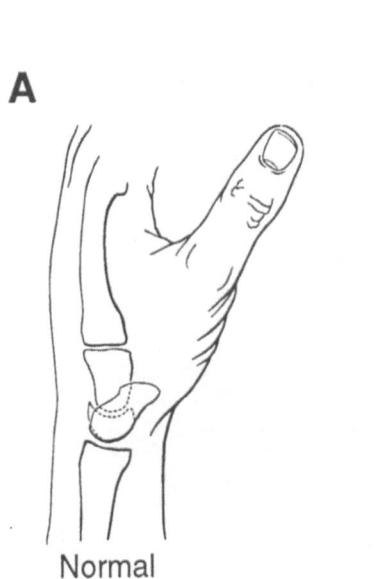

Normal

C

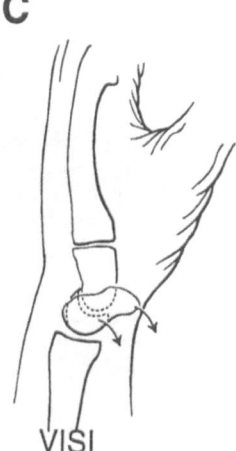

VISI

Fig. 5-4. A schematic diagram of the radius, capitate, lunate, scaphoid and second metacarpal bones (A) in their normal alignment, (B) with a Dorsal intercalated segment instability (DISI), and (C) with a Volar intercalated segment instability (VISI).

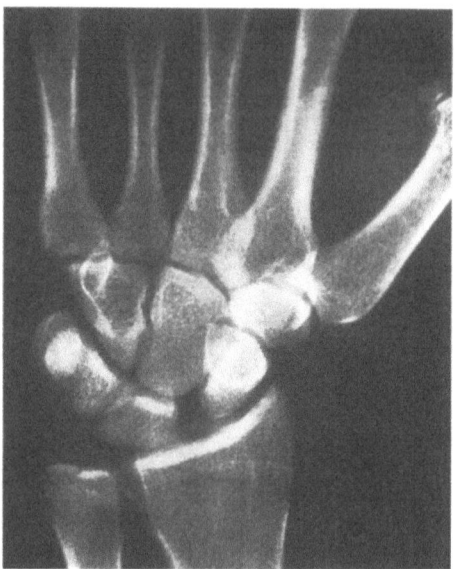

Fig. 5–5. An AP supinated clenched fist view of a wrist with a DISI deformity.

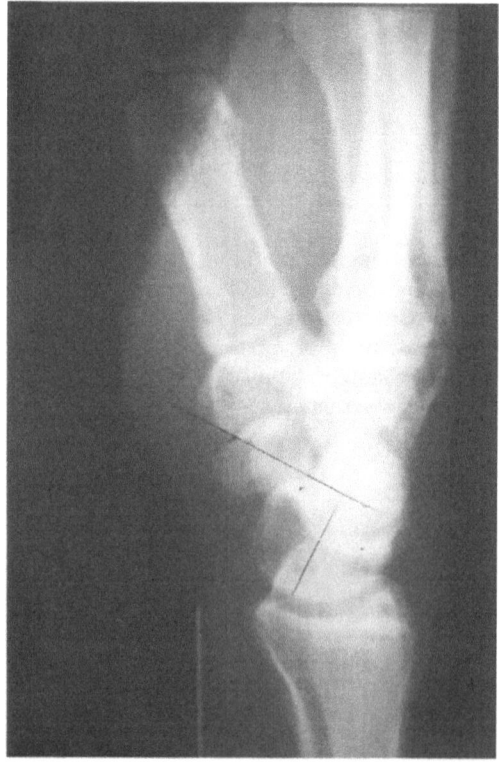

Fig. 5–6. A lateral radiograph of a wrist with a DISI deformity showing the flexed posture of the scaphoid and extended posture of the lunate.

general acceptance of the limited scaphoid trapezium trapezoid inter-carpal fusion for treatment of scapholunate dissociation with a DISI deformity. However, more recently, there are increasing questions regarding the complication rate and reliability of this procedure. Consideration is again being given to ligament repair/reconstruction of the scapholunate interosseous ligament.

If a scapholunate dissociation with a DISI deformity is not addressed, the natural history is believed to be progressive arthritis leading to a scapholunate advanced collapse (SLAC) wrist pattern of deformity (Figs. 5-7, 5-8). At one time, recommendations for treatment included excision of the scaphoid with placement of a silastic scaphoid implant. Problems with silastic synovitis have, in essence, resulted in the abandonment of this treatment for the SLAC wrist (Fig. 5-9). Although a limited carpal arthrodesis is currently a treatment option, this treatment still has some questions regarding long-term results. Complete wrist arthrodesis for a SLAC wrist remains an accepted treatment option.

Carpal dislocations and transcarpal fracture dislocations are significant injuries of the wrist. The mechanism for most of these injuries is a fall on an outstretched hand, with resultant hyperextension of the wrist with intercarpal supination. The lunate is considered the cornerstone of the carpus and is the carpal bone that has the most stabilizing ligaments to the forearm. Therefore, most injuries are of the perilunar type in which, for example, a dorsal perilunate dislocation will dislodge the entire carpus from the lunate, leaving the lunate still in the lunate fossa of the radius while the rest of the carpus dislocates dorsally (Fig. 5-10). A volar lunate dislocation results from further disruption of the dorsal capsule and ligamentous attachment to the lunate, allowing the lunate to flex forward, pivoting on its stronger volar ligaments, thereby allowing the perilunar carpus to reduce back onto the radius and ulna while the lunate is dislocated in a palmar direction. The pathognomonic radiographic shape of a volarly dislocated lunate is that of a triangle (Fig. 5-11). The treatment for a volar lunate dislocation is often described in the literature as a closed reduction followed by immobilization. However, due to the carpal instability from perilunar ligamentous disruption, there is a tendency for the lunate to assume an extension posture and the scaphoid to flex, resulting in a DISI deformity which cannot be reduced and held by closed immobilization. If carpal alignment is not anatomic on plane X-rays, or there is significant increase in the scapholunate gap (normally < 3 mm) and/or the scapholunate angle is abnormal (normally < 70° in a true lateral view), further measures need to be taken to accomplish an anatomic reduction and maintain that reduction. The goal of an anatomic reduction remains appropriate, even beyond the acute period of perilunar and lunate dislocations. Associated carpal fractures, either small avulsion fractures significant in demon-

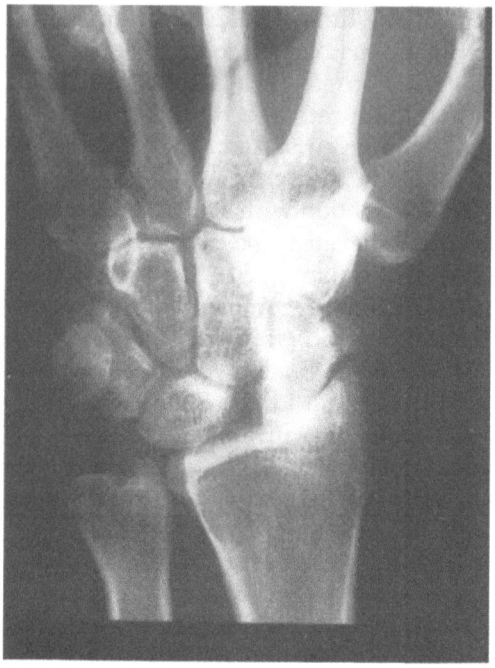

Fig. 5-7. A PA radiograph of a wrist with scapholunate advanced collapse (SLAC) showing decreased joint space between the scaphoid and radius, a widened scapholunate joint space, and some early narrowing between the capitate and the radial aspect of the lunate.

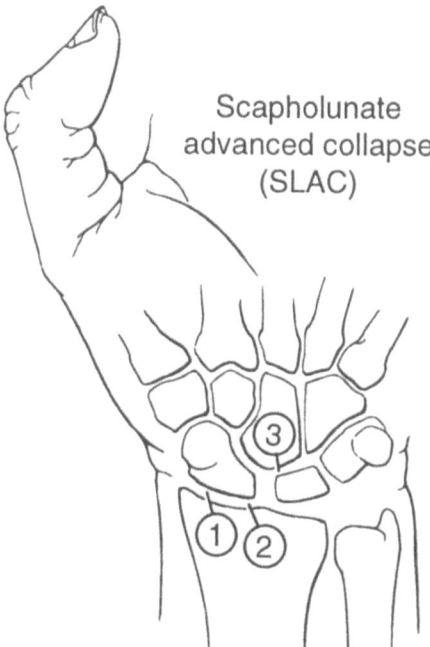

Scapholunate
advanced collapse
(SLAC)

Fig. 5-8. An illustration showing the progression of joint space narrowing and degenerative changes in a wrist that developed scapholunate advanced collapse. (1) Changes are first noted between the radial styloid and the scaphoid. (2) The changes then progress to involve the entire radioscaphoid joint. (3) Changes are seen between the radial aspect of the lunate and the proximal capitate. Final changes would be pancarpal arthritis.

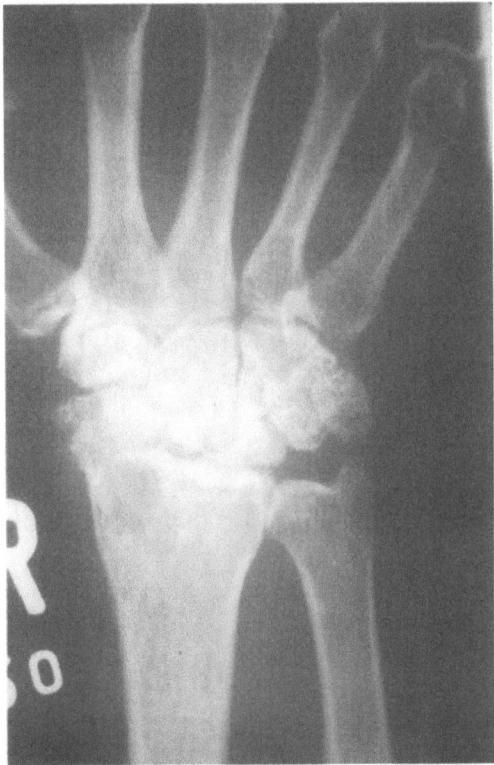

Fig. 5-9. A PA radiograph of a wrist (which has developed Silastic synovitis) showing inflammatory cystic changes, secondary to the inflammatory synovitis from the particulate debris of the silastic implant.

strating probable ligamentous disruption or scaphoid or other perilunar carpal fractures, or radial or ulnar styloid fractures, should be looked for on the plane X-rays to help diagnose and treat these carpal injuries. The overall alignment of the carpus in relation to the radius should also be assessed to identify any ulnar translation of the carpus which is a much more global instability, which perhaps may best be treated by radiolunate arthrodesis.

The scaphoid is the carpal bone that is most commonly fractured and has the highest incidence, compared to the other carpal bones, of nonunion following fracture (Fig. 5-12). This is due, in part, to its blood supply, which flows primarily from a distal to a proximal direction. A volar approach for open reduction and bone grafting of a scaphoid nonunion has been recommended because it is the least likely to injure the blood supply to the scaphoid. The more proximal the level of the scaphoid fracture, the greater the likelihood of nonunion, and the longer the period of immobilization should be. Generally, a distal tubercle

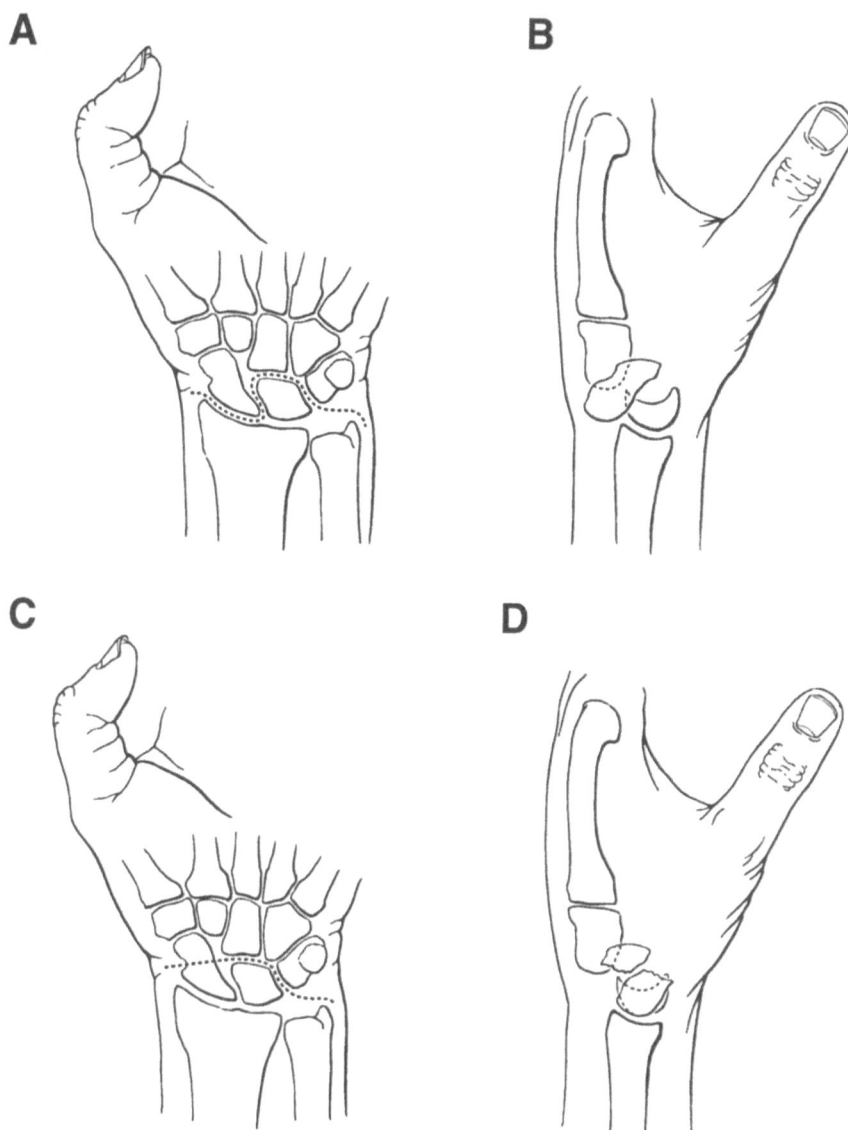

Fig. 5-10. Diagrammatic illustrations showing (A) the pattern of perilunar ligamentous disruption that can result in (B) a dorsal perilunate dislocation, and (C) the pattern of bone and ligamentous disruption that can result in (D) a dorsal transcaphoid perilunate fracture/dislocation.

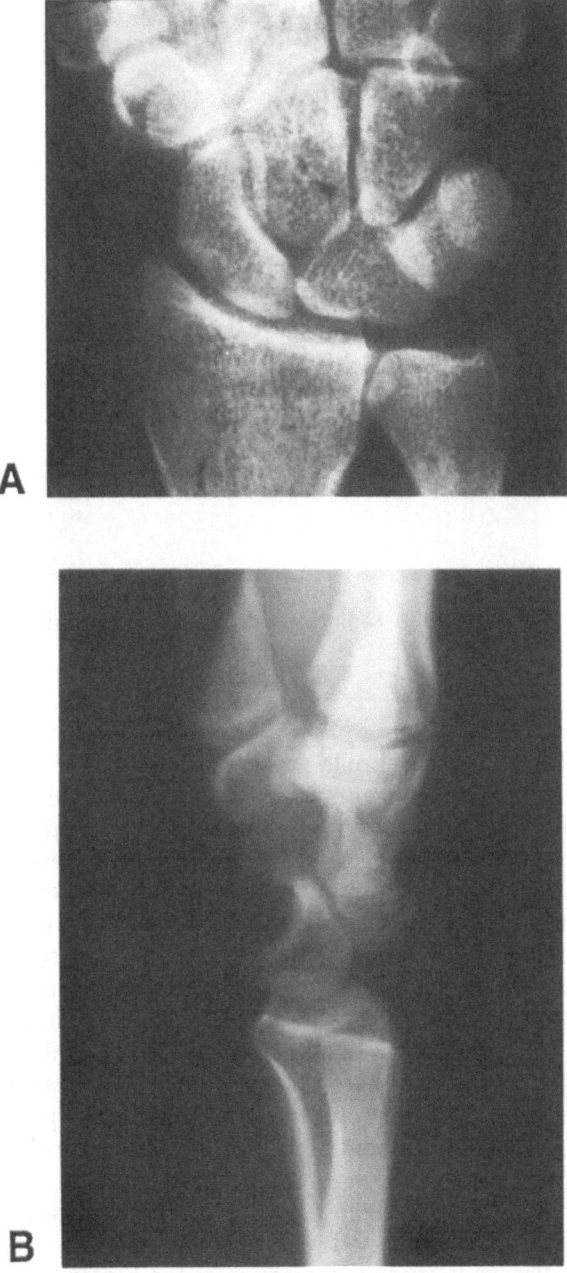

Fig. 5-11. (A) A PA radiograph showing the pathognomonic radiographic shape of a volarly dislocated lunate, which is that of a triangle. (B) The lateral radiograph readily shows the volarly dislocated lunate.

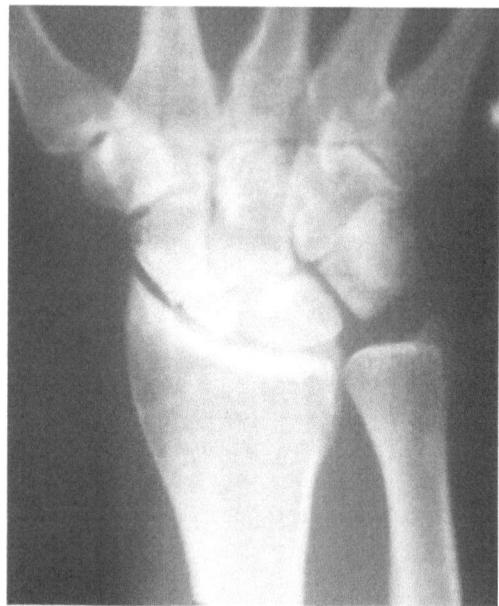

Fig. 5-12. A PA radiograph of a scaphoid fracture.

fracture of the scaphoid should be immobilized 4 to 6 weeks. A waist-level fracture of the scaphoid should be immobilized for 6 to 8 weeks. A proximal pole scaphoid fracture should be immobilized for 10 to 12 weeks. Delayed diagnosis and treatment of a scaphoid fracture increases the likelihood of a nonunion developing. Therefore, if a delay in diagnosis and treatment of a scaphoid fracture occurs, immobilization should include a long arm thumb spica cast, as opposed to the acute diagnosis and treatment of a scaphoid fracture, in which a short arm thumb spica cast is generally the accepted treatment. Closed treatment of a scaphoid fracture that is not acutely diagnosed is still an acceptable treatment approach, unless there is displacement of greater than 1 mm, cystic changes at the fracture site, and/or carpal malalignment. Treatment of an established scaphoid nonunion is autogenous bone grafting of the defect and postoperative immobilization.

Fracture of the pisiform which results in nonunion can be treated by surgical excision of the ununited pisiform.

Kienbock's disease is avascular necrosis of the lunate. In Caucasians, ulnar negative variance is commonly associated with Kienbock's disease. On plane X-rays, the relative increase in radiodensity seen in the lunate in Kienbock's disease is a result of increased osteoclastic activity in the surrounding carpus (Fig. 5-13). Early stages of Kienbock's disease

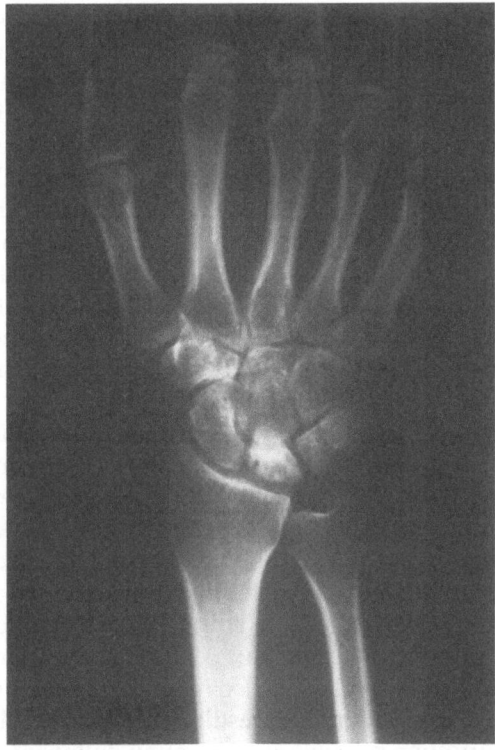

Fig. 5-13. A PA radiograph showing increased radiopacity of the lunate, compared to the surrounding carpus, in a patient with Kienbock's disease.

before significant lunate collapse, fragmentation, and carpal malalignment have been successfully treated with radial shortening or ulnar lengthening. In the event that a preadolescent child develops Kienbock's disease, a trial of cast immobilization may be an acceptable treatment approach. For the more severe stages of Kienbock's disease, proximal row carpectomy is a reasonable salvage option, and most cases will result in some decreased strength with good pain relief and functional wrist motion. At one time, an accepted treatment option for Kienbock's disease was excision of the lunate and insertion of a silastic lunate implant. Problems developed, however, with silastic synovitis. This condition would present with a synovitis and a limitation of motion. Radiographs could show fragmentation of the prosthesis with subchondral cysts in the radius and/or surrounding carpal bones. Treatment of silastic synovitis from carpal bone implants is generally a salvage procedure and includes synovectomy, debridement, removal of the implant, and wrist arthrodesis. Use of silastic carpal implants is no longer recommended.

Fracture of the distal radius is a common injury. Simple extraarticular fractures of the distal radius without significant comminution can often be adequately treated by closed reduction and immobilization with a cast. The brachioradialis is recognized to exert a deforming force on the distal radius fracture. The position of immobilization recommended to eliminate the effects of this deforming force is to immobilize the forearm in supination. In the event of significant comminution and/or deformity of the distal radius, additional measures to prevent persistent or recurring deformity of the radius are recommended. Previously, this type of treatment included pins and plaster immobilization. Currently, however, some type of external fixation is the generally accepted treatment. Intraarticular fracture step-off, gaping, and radial shortening are correlated with less optimal functional outcomes.

When a fracture of the distal radius involves the volar portion of the distal radius, the position of immobilization is recommended to be flexion. Distal radius volar intraarticular fractures often require open reduction and internal fixation of the fracture fragment.

There are a number of complications that can result from distal radius fractures. Arthrofibrosis, with resulting limited range of motion, can occur. Causes for this include a splint or cast that extends too far distally, thus blocking MP flexion. Postfracture swelling and loss of compliance of the dorsal skin can also result in limited flexion of the MP joint. Both of these situations can result in MCP joint collateral ligament contractures. Another possible complication following fracture of the distal radius, particularly with a volarly displaced bone fragment, is attritional rupture of one or more of the flexor tendons of the digits. Rupture of the extensor pollicis longus tendon can also occur following a distal radius fracture, even a nondisplaced distal radius fracture. An extensor pollicis longus tendon rupture can be treated by an extensor indicis proprius transfer or tendon graft. Swelling following a distal radius fracture, especially if there is a circumferential cast, can result in an increase in intracompartmental pressure and compartment syndrome. Whenever there is an open fracture and associated soft tissue trauma, infection is a concern, and treatment of the fracture with an external fixator offers a better opportunity to assess the wound and perform local wound care.

Distal radius fractures in the child with open growth plates may result in premature complete or partial epiphyseal closure.

The triangular fibrocartilage complex, consisting of the central triangular fibrocartilage and a dorsal and volar radioulnar ligament, is the major contribution to the static stability of the distal radioulnar joint. Although there has been some discrepancy in the literature, now the generally accepted opinion is that disruption of the dorsal radioulnar ligament results in instability dorsally, with a more prominent distal ulna with forearm pronation. This is best treated by immobilization with the forearm in supination. Disruption of the palmar radioulnar ligament results in a more prominent ulnar head with the forearm supinated, and is best reduced with the forearm in full pronation.

Recommended Reading

Cooney, W. P. III, J. H. Dobyns, annd R. L. Linscheid. 1980. Fractures of the scaphoid: a rational approach to management. Clin. Orthop. Rel. Res. 149:90.

Cooney, W.P., E. L. Linscheid and J. H. Dobyns. 1992. Carpal instability: treatment of ligament injuries of the wrist. Instructional Course Lectures 41:33.

Gelberman, R.H., and J. Menon. 1980. The vascularity of the scaphoid bone. J. Hand Surg. 5:508.

Levinsohn, E. M., I. D. Rosen, and A. H. Palmer. 1991. Wrist arthrography: value of the three-compartment injection method. Radiology 179:231.

Linscheid, R. L., J. H. Dobyns, J. W. Beabout, and R. S. Bryan. 1972. Traumatic instability of the wrist: diagnosis, classification, and pathomechanics. J. Bone Joint Surg. 54:1612.

Mayfield, J. K., R. P. Johnson, and R. K. Kilcoyne. 1980. Carpal dislocations: pathomechanics and progressive perilunar instability. J. Hand Surg. 5:226.

Palmer, A. K. 1993. Fractures of the distal radius. *In:* Operative hand surgery, 3rd Ed., ed. D. P. Green, 929. New York: Churchill Livingstone.

Trumble, T. E., S. R. Schmitt, and N. B. Vedder. 1994. Factors affecting functional outcome of displaced intra-articular distal radius fractures. J. Hand Surg. 19A:325.

Viegas, S. F. 1994. Carpal instabilities. *In:* Hand surgery update, Chap. 10, 1–13. American Society for Surgery of the Hand, Englewood, Co.

Questions

A. After falling on his outstretched hand, a 23-year-old male is found on a lateral X-ray of the wrist to have the axis of the scaphoid 47° volar to the axis of the lunate (a 47° scapholunate angle). This finding would suggest:

1. Lunate dislocation
2. Perilunar dislocation
3. Volar rotary subluxation of the scaphoid
4. Dorsal rotary subluxation of the scaphoid
5. Normal scapholunate alignment

B. A 28-year-old male involved in a motorcycle accident injures his left wrist. The radiograph (Fig. 5–14) shows a dislocated:

1. Lunate
2. Scaphoid
3. Lunate and pisiform
4. Lunate and fractured radial styloid
5. Lunate and fractured scaphoid

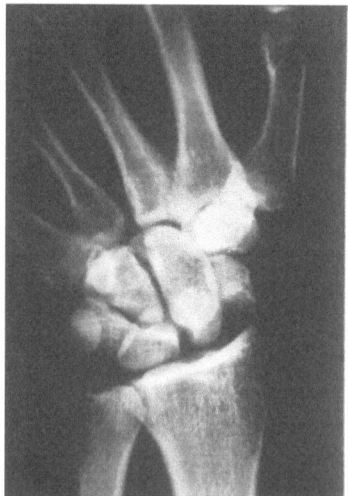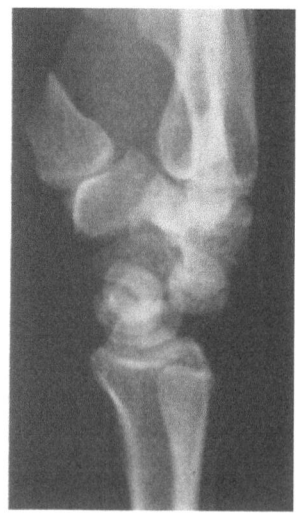

Fig. 5–14.

C. Figure 5–15 shows the radiographic appearance of the dominant wrist of a 22-year-old laborer following 7 months of cast immobilization. Your treatment would be to:

1. Remove the cast and return to work
2. Remove the cast and refer to physical therapy
3. Insert autogenous bone graft and immobilize in a cast
4. Insert a scaphoid compression screw
5. Replace the scaphoid with a silastic prosthesis

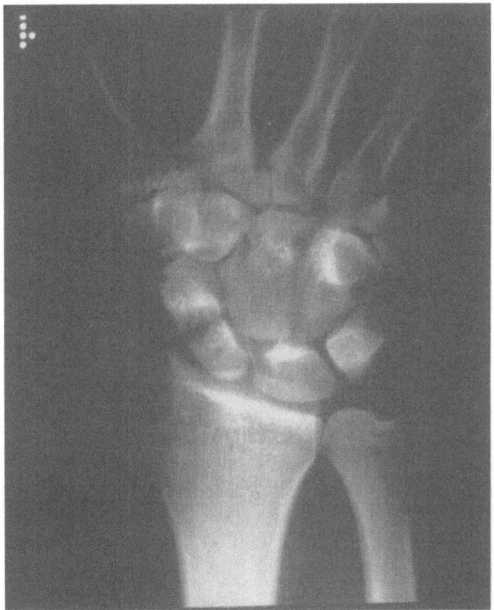

Fig. 5–15.

D. Figure 5-16 shows the radiograph of an 18-year-old high school gymnast who has had some pain in her wrist for the past 8 months. The patient has not been taking any medications. Physical examination reveals tenderness over the dorsal aspect of her wrist, and the range of motion in her wrist is 75% of that in her other wrist. The patient's wrist pain is most likely caused by:

1. Scapholunate instability
2. Lunotriquetral dissociation
3. A stress fracture
4. Juvenile rheumatoid arthritis
5. Necrosis of the lunate

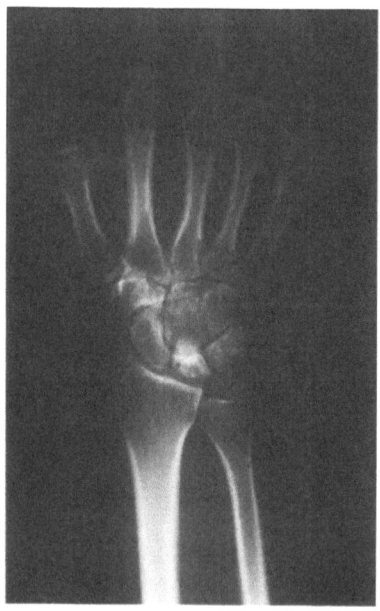

Fig. 5-16.

E. Which among the components of deformity in an extraarticular distal radius fracture is most important to restore for obtaining a satisfactory outcome after closed reduction of an extraarticular distal radius fracture?

1. Radial inclination
2. Radial translation
3. Radial length
4. Palmar tilt
5. Pronation/supination

F. A 63-year-old woman notices the recent inability to straighten her thumb and the development of pain over the dorsum of the wrist 4 months after she had healed a distal radius fracture (Colles'). Examination revealed an inability to actively extend the IP joint of the thumb and tenderness over the dorsal distal wrist. Radiographs demonstrate a healed Colles' fracture in good alignment. Her most likely diagnosis is:

1. Flexor pollicis longus tendinitis
2. Extensor tendinitis
3. Extensor pollicis longus rupture
4. Posttraumatic arthritis
5. Posterior interosseous nerve compression

G. A six-year-old boy sustained a closed greenstick fracture of the distal right forearm 3 months earlier. The patient was treated at another facility with a closed reduction. The fracture of the distal end of the radius and ulna healed without evidence of physeal or epiphyseal injury. Radiographs now show there is a deformity of the distal radius and ulna with apex volar angulation of 30°, 3 cm proximal to the physis. Without further treatment, you would anticipate:

1. The same volar angulation
2. Some improvement in the volar deviation
3. A short forearm
4. A normal forearm
5. Arthritis of the wrist joint

6 Tumors

The most common tumor of the hand is actually a ganglion cyst. The most common location of a ganglion cyst in the hand is at the dorsal aspect of the wrist. The common site of origin for the stalk of a dorsal wrist ganglion is the dorsal aspect of the scapholunate interosseous ligament (Fig. 6–1). Ganglion cysts can also be commonly seen at the dorsal radial or dorsal ulnar aspect of the DIP joints of the fingers. This is sometimes called a mucinous cyst and is most often associated with osteoarthritis. Treatment of these mucinous cysts, which can result in thinning of the overlying skin and deformity of the nail, can include cyst excision, joint debridement, and skin coverage or, alternatively, arthrodesis of the DIP joint.

Myositis ossificans can develop following an injury or trauma and typically involves the brachialis muscle at the anterior aspect of the elbow, resulting in a firmly fixed mass and limited motion of the elbow. The most pertinent histologic features that will assist in making the diagnosis are a more mature zone of bone peripherally in the lesion with immature bone and cellular elements centrally. Treatment for myositis ossificans is generally observation and gentle active range of motion.

The supracondylar process of the humerus, which is found in approximately 1% of the population, is an anomalous bony spur of variable size located 3 to 5 cm proximal to the elbow on the anterior medial aspect of the humerus (Fig. 6–2). The supracondylar process, if present, can often be palpated. The range of motion of the elbow should not be limited, and the patient should have no symptomatic or functional complaints related to the supracondylar process in the upper extremity. Medial displacement of the median nerve is an anatomic variation that can be seen in association with a supracondylar process of the humerus. Treatment is merely observation, although median nerve symptoms may occasionally be associated with the presence of a supracondylar process of the humerus.

Malignant tumors below the elbow are rare. The most common malignant tumor of the hand is the squamous cell carcinoma. Treatment

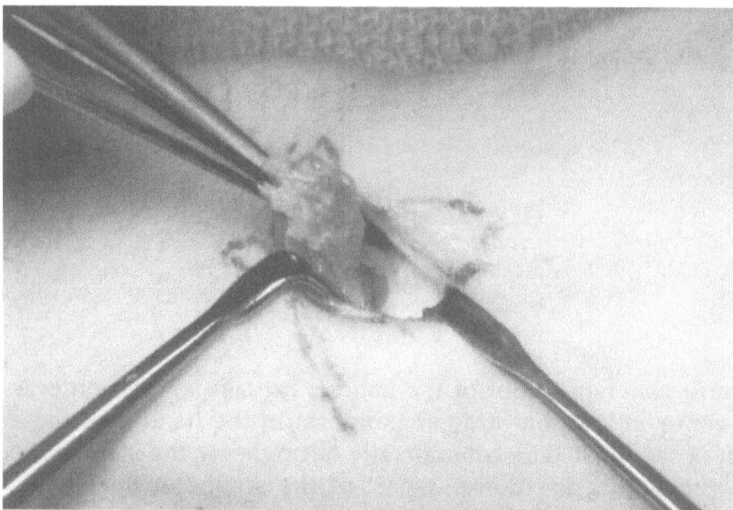

Fig. 6-1. An intraoperative photograph showing a dorsal wrist ganglion with the stalk originating from the scapholunate interosseous ligament.

of squamous cell carcinoma is surgical excision, which should include a wide margin.

The most common soft tissue sarcoma of the hand is the epithelioid sarcoma. Other soft tissue malignant tumors found in the upper extremity are synovial sarcoma, Ewing's tumor, and osteogenic sarcoma. Treatment of these tumors should also be surgical excision, including a wide margin. When one of these tumors involves a digit, the digit should be amputated and, depending on the size and location of the lesion, this excision may need to include a ray resection and/or subtotal amputation of the hand and possible axillary node dissection.

The most common bone tumor of the hand is an enchondroma. Patients with enchondromas may present with symptoms of pain. The pain is associated with a fracture of the thinned cortical margin resulting from the expanding enchondroma. The presentation of patients with an enchondroma, in fact, is often for evaluation of a pathologic fracture through the lesion. In that case, the most appropriate treatment is curettage and bone grafting after the fracture has healed. In the event that there is no pathologic fracture, bone grafting following curettage is considered the treatment of choice. A patient presenting with multiple enchondromatosis can have multiple lesions of the hand, including painless shortening or deformity of the forearm and hand.

A giant cell tumor of bone can occur in the upper extremity. Two of the most common locations for a giant cell tumor of bone are the distal radius and the distal ulna. The radiographic appearance of the lesion is typically lytic in nature and expanding. If sufficiently large, there can be

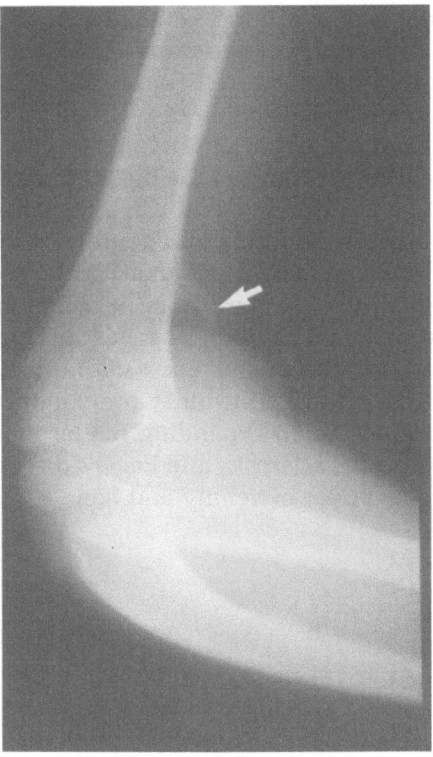

Fig. 6–2. A radiograph of a humerus with a supracondylar process (arrow) at its anterior medial border, proximal to the medial epicondyle.

cortical thinning and even defects in the cortex. The giant cell tumor is one of the few lesions that can cross the growth plate, the others being a chondroblastoma and a brown tumor of hyperparathyroidism. The histology of a giant cell tumor will typically include multiple giant cells, of which the nuclei look the same as the nuclei of the surrounding cells. Depending on the size of the lesion and integrity of the cortical bone, aggressive curettement and autogenous bone grafting or filling of the defect with methyl methacrylate have been recommended or, alternatively, block excision of the distal radius or ulna with bone grafting. Giant cell tumors of the hand have been reported to have a more aggressive history; because of this tendency, more aggressive surgical treatment has been recommended.

Aneurysmal bone cysts may have a somewhat similar appearance radiographically to the giant cell tumor of bone. It may also have, on histology, giant cells, although the nuclei of the giant cells in an aneurysmal bone cyst are dissimilar from the surrounding cell nuclei.

Juxtacortical chondromas can also occur in the hand, and treatment can include local excision and bone grafting. Benign fibromatosis has also been identified in the upper extremity.

A neurilemmoma, or Schwann cell tumor, is a benign nerve lesion and treatment should include excision of the tumor with sparing of the nerve fascicles. A giant cell tumor of tendon sheath is one of the more common soft tissue benign tumors of the digits. Lipomas can also occur in the hand and upper extremity and can arise in an intramuscular location or within a nerve, resulting in a neurolipofibroma.

A hemangioma is a vascular tumor that can be seen in the upper extremity. A patient with a hemangioma, if symptomatic, can notice increased symptoms coinciding with changes in blood flow, such as during exposure to temperature changes and/or exertion.

An aneurysm or thrombosis of the ulnar artery in the hypothenar area of the hand can present as an expanding tender mass. Gouty tophi, fibrous dysplasia, tuberous sclerosis, and Paget's disease can all result in masses in the hand or upper extremity and bone lesions on X-rays.

Recommended Reading

Al Qattan, M. M., and J. B. Husband. 1991. Median nerve compression by the supracondylar process: a case report. J. Hand Surg. 16B:101.

Averill, R. M., R. J. Smith, and C. J. Campbell. 1980. Giant cell tumor of the bones of the hand. J. Hand Surg. 5:39.

Bryan, R. S., E. H. Soule, and J. H. Dobyns. 1974. Primary epithelioid sarcoma of the hand and forearm: a review of thirteen cases. J. Bone Joint Surg. 56A:458.

Creighton, J. J., C. A. Peimer, E. R. Mindell, D. C. Boone, C. P. Karakonis, and H. O. Douglass. 1985. Primary malignant tumors of the upper extremity: retrospective analysis of 126 cases. J. Hand Surg. 10A:805.

Enzinger, F. M., and S. W. Weiss. 1983. Soft tissue tumors. St Louis: Mosby.

Greenspan, A. 1989. Tumors of cartilage origin. Orthop. Clin. North Am. 20:247.

Mankin, H. J. 1987. Principles of diagnosis and management of tumors of the hand. Hand Clin. 3:185.

Peimer, C. A., O. J. Moy, and H. M. Dick. 1993. Tumors of bone and soft tissue. In: Operative hand surgery, 3rd Ed., ed. D. P. Green, 2225. New York: Churchill Livingstone.

Rydholm, A., and N. O. Berg. 1983. Size, site, and clinical incidence of lipomas: factors in differential diagnosis of lipoma and sarcoma. Acta Orthop. Scand. 54:929.

Questions

A. The dorsal wrist ganglion most commonly originates from the:

1. Extensor carpi radialis brevis tendon sheath
2. Radiocarpal joint capsule
3. Second carpometacarpal joint capsule
4. Scapholunate ligament
5. Lunotriquetral ligament

B. A 16-year-old football player fell on his left arm 5 weeks ago. He has had pain and his right elbow motion has become increasingly limited. X-rays of the lesion are shown in Figure 6–3a. Photomicrographs from a biopsy of the tissue are shown in Figures 6–3b and c (see color insert). The diagnosis is:

1. Osteosarcoma
2. Osteoblastoma
3. Myositis ossificans
4. Polymyositis
5. Heterotopic ossification

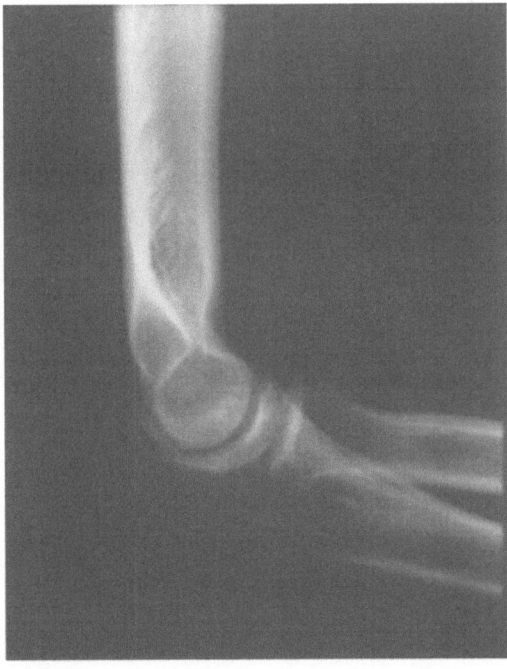

Fig. 6–3a.

C. A mother brings in her 6-year-old boy for assessment of a bump she first noticed in his arm just proximal to the elbow several weeks ago, which has persisted but has not changed in size since he first noticed it several weeks ago. Examination shows a palpable, firm swelling just proximal to the medial aspect of his elbow joint. X-rays are shown in Figure 6-4. Initial management should consist of:

1. A CT scan
2. An MRI
3. An arteriogram
4. Excisional biopsy
5. Observation

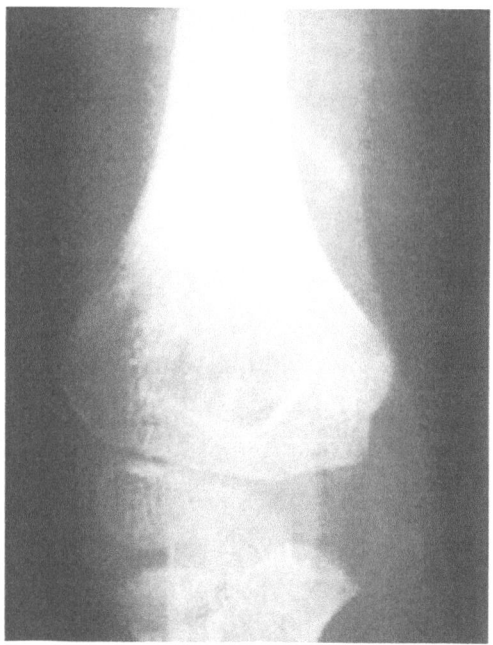

Fig. 6-4.

D. A 67-year-old farmer presented with the lesion shown in Figure 6–5a on his dominant index finger. A PA radiograph is seen in Figure 6–5b. A biopsy of the finger is seen in Figures 6–5c and d (see color insert). A metastatic workup showed no evidence of any other lesion. Treatment should be:

1. Local excision, skeletal shortening, and primary closure
2. Wide local excision and split-thickness skin grafting
3. Disarticulation at the metacarpophalangeal joint
4. Ray resection
5. Amputation of the hand and axillary node dissection

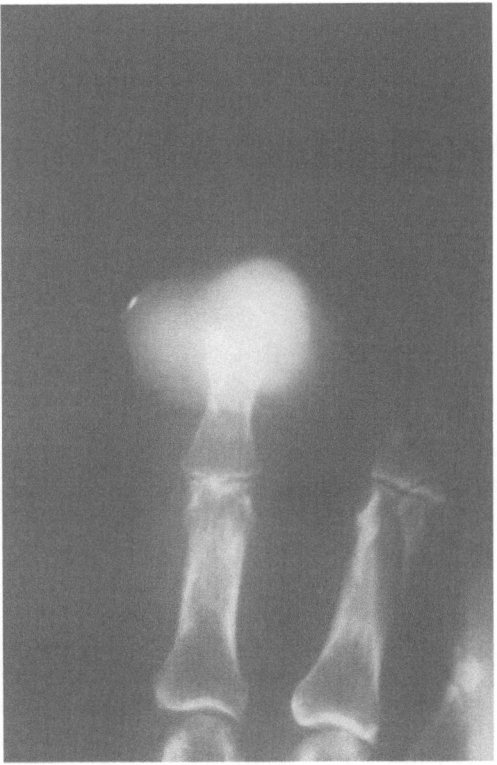

Fig. 6–5b.

E. Epithelioid sarcoma in the distal aspect of the right index finger in a 32-year-old concert pianist should be treated by:

1. Local excision skeletal shortening and primary closure
2. Wide resection and a skin flap
3. Irradiation
4. Index ray resection
5. Below-the-elbow amputation

F. Figure 6–6a shows the radiographs of a painful digit of a 23-year-old saleswoman. A biopsy of the digit is seen in Figures 6–6b and c. The lesion requires:

1. Observation
2. Irradiation
3. Ray resection
4. Chemotherapy and wide resection
5. Curettage and bone grafting

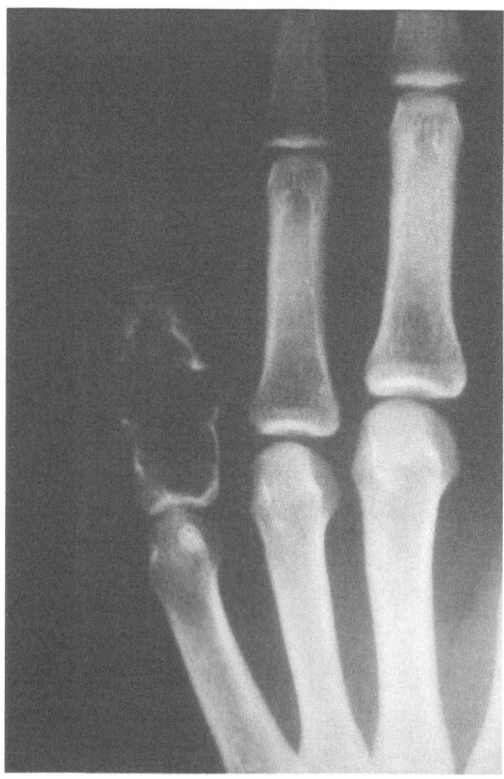

Fig. 6–6a.

Color Plates

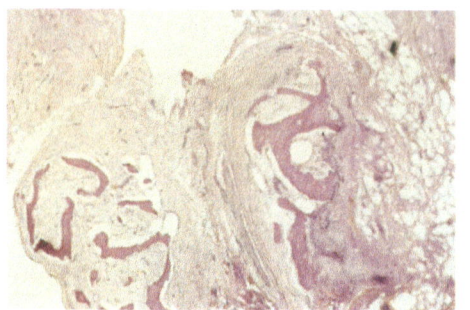

Fig. 6-3b

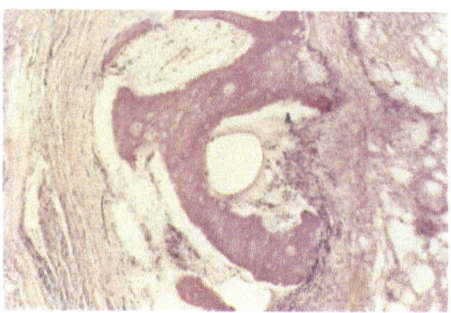

Fig. 6-3c

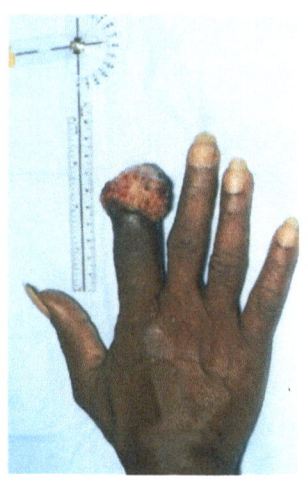

Fig. 6-5a

Fig. 6-5c

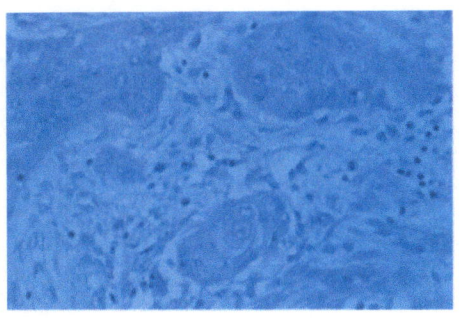

Fig. 6-5d

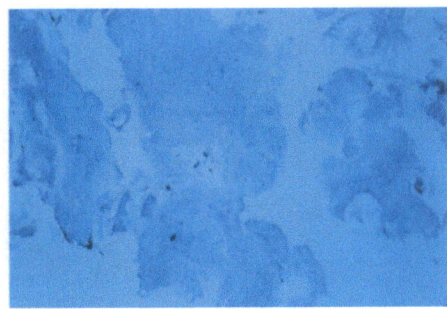

Fig. 6-6b

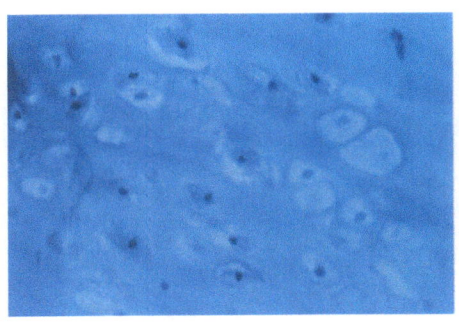

Fig. 6-6c

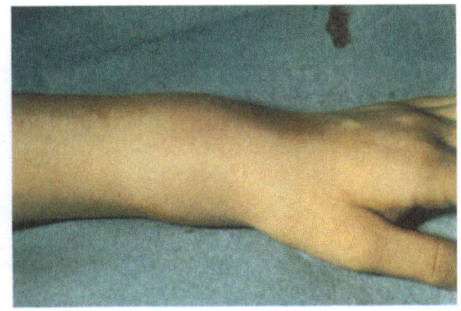

Fig. 6-7a

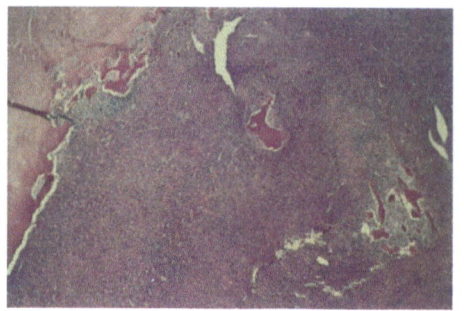

Fig. 6-7d

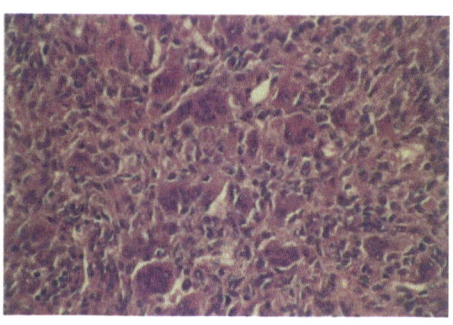

Fig. 6-7e

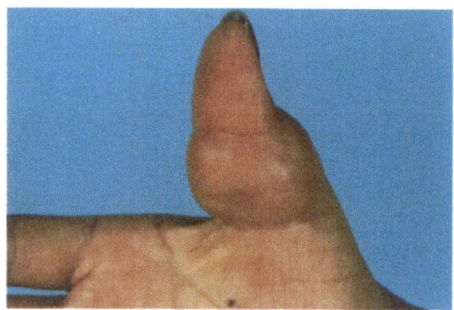

Fig. 6-8a

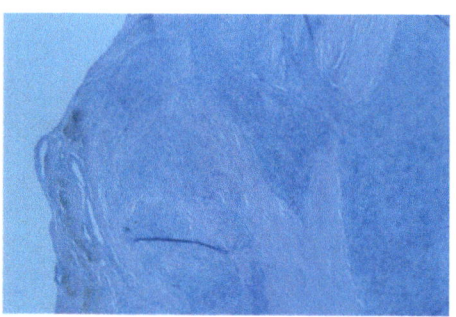

Fig. 6-8b

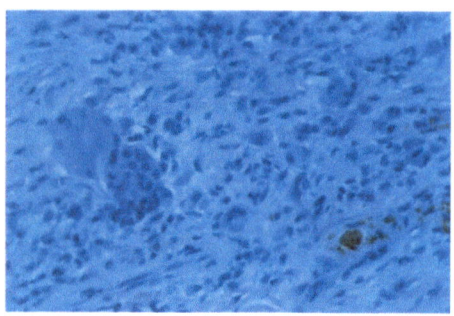

Fig. 6-8c

G. A 25-year-old female has 3 months of pain and swelling in her right wrist (Fig. 6–7a; see color insert). The roentgenogram is shown in Figure 6–7b. An MRI is shown in Figure 6–7c. Laboratory values are normal. The biopsy is shown in Figure 6–7d and e (see color insert). This represents:

1. A giant cell tumor of bone
2. A brown tumor of hyperparathyroidism
3. A nonossifying fibroma
4. A tuberculous osteomyelitis
5. A metastatic thymoma

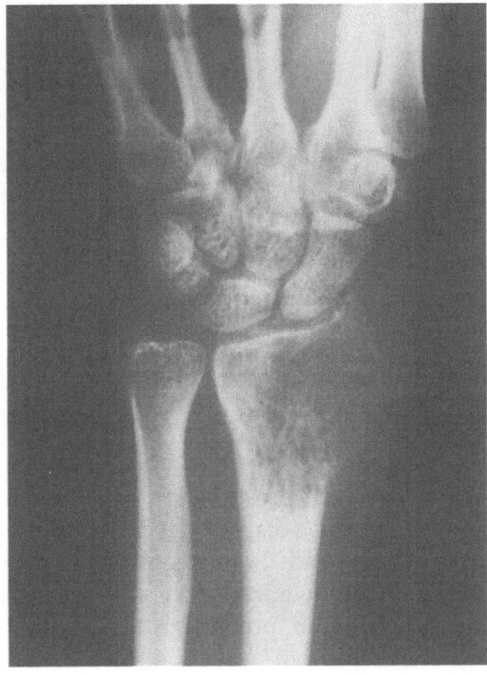

Fig. 6–7b.

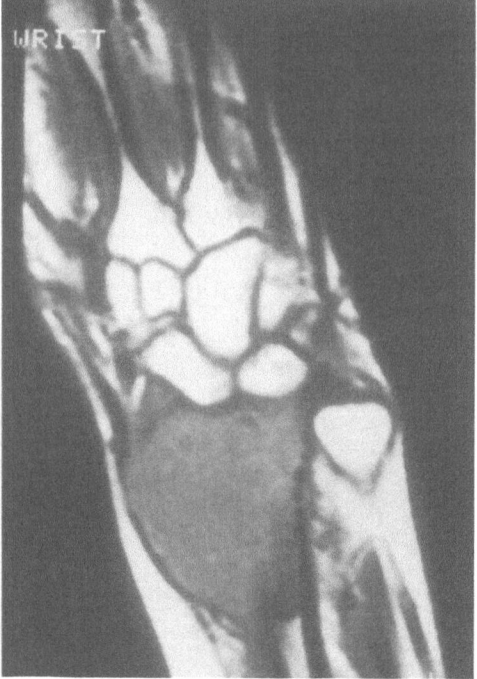

Fig. 6–7c.

H. A 35-year-old male has a 1.5-cm neurilemmoma of the median nerve at the wrist. Treatment should be:

1. Below-elbow amputation
2. Excision of the tumor with preservation of all nerve fascicles
3. Excision of the tumor and adjacent nerve fascicles
4. Excision of the tumor and 2-cm segment of proximal and distal median nerve, followed by sural nerve graft of the defect
5. Excision of the tumor and involved nerve with mobilization and primary repair of the median nerve

I. A 25-year-old woman presents with a slowly enlarging nontender mass in her right thumb (Fig. 6–8a; see color insert). Radiographs do not show any bone changes. Photomicrographs of the lesion are shown in Figures 6–8b and c (see color insert). The most likely diagnosis is:

1. Epidermal inclusion cyst
2. Ganglion cyst
3. Foreign body granuloma
4. Giant cell tumor of tendon sheath
5. Fibrosarcoma

7 Nerve Injuries

General Peripheral

Electrical evidence of denervation following a nerve injury first appears at approximately 3 weeks following the injury. Spontaneous fibrillations will first appear in denervated muscle following transection of the motor axon approximately 2 to 4 weeks following the nerve injury. Axonal growth following primary repair of a peripheral nerve laceration occurs at a rate of 1 mm/day after an initial period of postinjury repair.

One of the most important prognostic factors in the recovery of a peripheral nerve following repair of a complete laceration is the age of the patient. Somatic motor nerve fibers have the greatest diameter and the greatest conduction velocities. Pain perception is the last function to be compromised in a nerve that is under pressure for an extended period of time. Mechanical deformation in a compressive neuropathy of a peripheral nerve has been found to be greatest in the superficial regions of the nerve and in the zones between compressed and uncompressed segments of the nerve.

A positive Tinel's sign can be a clinical indication that nerve regeneration is occurring, and continued migration of the Tinel's sign distal from the site of anastomosis of a peripheral nerve laceration can indicate continued regeneration of that nerve. In a contaminated and/or dirty wound, repair of a nerve injury should be delayed generally 7 to 10 days. The sural nerve is generally considered the best choice for a donor nerve for grafting. If possible, treatment of a neuroma with a complete sensory deficit, such as in a radial sensory nerve, can be treated well by repair or grafting of the transected nerve. If there is a clean laceration of tendons and nerve, the recommended treatment is generally repair of the nerve and tendons primarily.

Recommended Reading

Gelberman, R. H., R. G. Eaton, and J. R. Urbaniak. 1994. Peripheral nerve compression. *In:* Instructional course lectures, XXXIII, ed. M. Schafer, 31. Rosemont, IL: American Academy of Orthopaedic Surgeons.

Lenman, J. A. R. and A. E. Ritchie. 1970. Clinical electromyography. Philadelphia: J.B. Lippincott Co.

Lundborg, G., B. Rydevik, M. Manthorpe, et al. 1988. Peripheral nerve: the physiology of injury and repair. *In:* Injury and repair of the musculoskeletal soft tissues, ed. S. L.-Y. Woo and J. A. Buckwalter, 297. Park Ridge, IL: American Academy of Orthopaedic Surgeons.

Van Beek, A. L., and P. Heyman. 1991. Electrophysiological testing. *In:* Operative nerve repair and reconstruction, ed. R. H. Gelberman, 171. Philadelphia: J.B. Lippincott Co.

Wilgis, E. F. S. and T. M. Brushart. 1993. Nerve repair and grafting. *In:* Operative hand surgery, 3rd Ed., ed. D. P. Green, 1315. New York: Churchill Livingstone.

Questions

A. Following complete laceration of a motor nerve, spontaneous fibrillations first appear in the denervated muscle:

1. Immediately
2. After 2 to 4 hours
3. After 2 to 4 days
4. After 2 to 4 weeks
5. After 2 to 4 months

B. The most important prognostic factor in the recovery of a complete laceration of a peripheral nerve just proximal to the wrist following surgical repair is:

1. Surgical repair 3 days or less following the injury
2. The patient's age
3. Repair of the nerve using visual magnification
4. Fascicular repair
5. The integrity of the associated artery

C. What neural structures develop the most mechanical deformation in a compressive neuropathy of a peripheral nerve?

1. Sympathetic nerves
2. Nerve segments between the nodes of Ranvier
3. Mixed motor and sensory nerves
4. Superficial regions of the nerve in areas between compressed and uncompressed segments of the nerve
5. Deeper regions of the nerve in areas between compressed and uncompressed segments of the nerve

Ulnar Nerve

A patient with a low ulnar nerve laceration at the level of the hypothenar eminence would have difficulty in turning a key in a tight lock. This weakness in pinch is noticed clinically when a patient compensates for this weakness and uses primarily the flexor pollicis longus to compensate for the weakened pinch and flexes the interphalangeal joint of the thumb against the flexed interphalangeal joint of the index finger in an opposed position. This maneuver is called the Froment's sign (Fig. 7–1). Another clinical finding in a patient with a low ulnar nerve palsy is the Wartenberg's sign, which is persistent abduction of the extended little finger due to the activity of the extensor digiti minimi, which is unopposed owing to the paralyzed third palmar interosseous muscle. Weakness in pinch and grip strength is largely due to loss of the adductor pollicis and first dorsal interosseous muscles.

A patient with a low ulnar nerve palsy may also demonstrate clawing of the ring and little fingers. This deformity is called an intrinsic minus posture. If a low median and ulnar nerve palsy exists, the index and long fingers, as well as the ring and little fingers, can all assume an intrinsic minus posture. Clawing is most likely to occur during attempted active extension of the ring and little fingers if the ulnar nerve lesion occurs at the level of the volar branch of the ulnar nerve at the

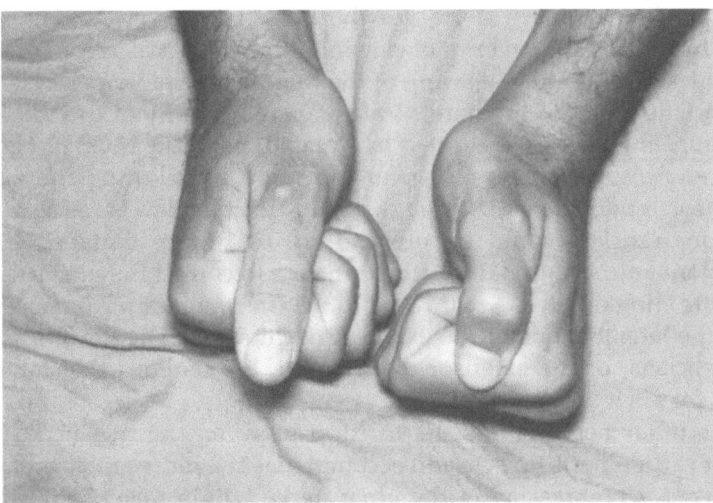

Fig. 7–1. A clinical photograph of a patient with a left hand ulnar nerve palsy, which results in weakness of the adductor muscle of the thumb. The flexor pollicis longus is used to compensate for the weakened pinch strength, and the IP joint is noted to assume a flexed posture. This maneuver is the Froment's sign.

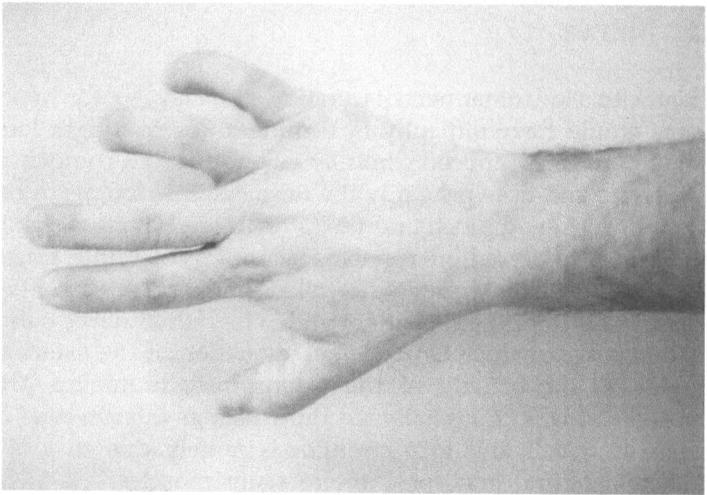

Fig. 7-2. A clinical photograph of an individual with a low ulnar nerve palsy who is attempting to extend his fingers. Due to loss of the intrinsic muscles to the little and ring fingers, the MP joint assumes a hyperextended posture, while the IP joints assume a flexed position. This is described as an intrinsic minus posture of the ring and little fingers and/or clawing of those digits.

wrist (Fig. 7-2). In high ulnar nerve palsy, clawing of the ring and little fingers is less pronounced because the flexor digitorum profundi are also paralyzed, which decreases the flexion force on the fingers and thereby lessens the severity of clawing. Many surgical procedures have been described to treat clawing of the fingers caused by paralysis of the intrinsic muscles of the hand. Volar capsulorrhaphy of the metacarpal phalangeal joints, as described by Zancoli, prevents MCP hyperextension and also improves PIP joint extension by allowing the extrinsic extensor tendon to pull through to the IP joint levels. Alternatively, tendon transfers could be used to try to restore dynamic intrinsic function; and, if this is done, the transfers to correct the intrinsic minus posture should follow a path volar to the transmetacarpal ligaments and into the lateral bands of the extensor mechanism. The flexor digitorum superficialis, or the extensor digiti quinti, are tendons that have been used for such a transfer.

The ulnar nerve enters the forearm between the two heads of the flexor carpi ulnaris muscle and accompanies the ulnar artery and vein at the wrist. Compression of the ulnar nerve within the cubital tunnel at the elbow can be treated by surgical transposition of the nerve anterior to the medial epicondyle. In performing the anterior transposition of the ulnar nerve, one must be careful to avoid injury to the medial antebrachial sensory nerve. Aneurysm of the ulnar artery and/or thrombosis of the ulnar artery in Guyon's canal can cause an ulnar neuropathy, due to the proximity of the ulnar artery and nerve in this location. Internal neurolysis of the ulnar or any other of the nerves has the highest likelihood of compromise to its blood supply and subsequent scarring. The dorsal cutaneous branch of the ulnar nerve supplies the dorsal ulnar surface of the hand and dorsal surface of the proximal phalanges of the middle and ring fingers.

Fracture of the lateral condyle of the humerus in childhood with subsequent displacement or growth arrest, resulting in a cubitus valgus deformity, can result in a tardy ulnar nerve palsy. This may present with weakness of the flexor digitorum profundus of the little and ring fingers, as well as weakness of the hypothenar muscles and intrinsics and decreased sensation of the little and ring fingers. Sufficient involvement may also result in some weakness of the flexor carpi ulnaris muscle. Elbow injuries that include injury to the medial collateral ligament may also have an ulnar neuropathy.

Recommended Reading

Anomer, G. E. 1993. Ulnar nerve palsy. *In:* Operative hand surgery, 3rd Ed., ed. D. P. Green, 1449. New York: Churchill Livingstone.

Eversmann, W. W. 1993. Entrapment in compression neuropathies. *In:* Operative hand surgery, 3rd Ed., ed. D. P. Green, 1356. New York: Churchill Livingstone.

Froimson, A. I., and F. Zahrawi. 1980. Treatment of compression neuropathy of the ulnar nerve at the elbow by epicondylectomy and neurolysis. J.Hand Surg. 5:391.

Masear, V. R., R. D. Meyer, and D. R. Pichora. 1989. Surgical anatomy of the medial antebrachial cutaneous nerve. J. Hand Surg. 14A:267.

Shea, J. D., and E. J. McClain. 1969. Ulnar-nerve compression syndromes at and below the wrist. J. Bone Joint Surg. 51A:1095.

Questions

A. A 25-year-old man lacerates the hypothenar eminence of his right hand with a clean knife and loses function of the deep branch of the ulnar nerve. He will notice loss of function of this nerve most when he tries to:

1. Hold a toothbrush
2. Hold a tennis ball
3. Pick up small pins
4. Carry a briefcase
5. Turn a key in a tight lock

B. A patient presents complaining of difficulty grasping things. The patient complains of weakness while trying to pull some paper from the physician's hand. The physician notices that he hyperflexes his thumb IP joint when he tries to pull at the paper. The patient is demonstrating a sign often seen with:

1. Radial nerve palsy
2. Posterior interosseous nerve palsy
3. Median nerve palsy
4. Ulnar nerve palsy
5. Extensor pollicis longus rupture

C. A patient would be most likely to demonstrate severe clawing of the ring and small fingers when he attempted to actively extend the fingers if he had an ulnar nerve lesion at the:

1. Roots contributing to the ulnar nerve from the brachial plexus
2. Midhumeral level
3. Elbow level
4. Volar branch of the ulnar nerve at the wrist
5. Dorsal branch of the ulnar nerve at the wrist

D. A patient has an ulnar nerve palsy and clawing of the ring finger and little finger. If the ring finger sublimis tendon is transferred to correct the deformity, the transfer must pass:

1. Volar to the transverse carpal ligament
2. Volar to the transverse intermetacarpal ligament
3. Dorsal to the center of rotation of the metacarpophalangeal joint
4. Volar to the center of rotation of the proximal interphalangeal joint
5. Ulnar to the metacarpophalangeal joint of the little finger

Radial Nerve

The radial nerve can be injured as a result of different types of trauma, including lacerations, blunt trauma, and distal humeral fractures. When the radial nerve is injured as a result of trauma that has also caused a closed fracture of the distal half of the humerus, the likelihood of spontaneous recovery of the radial nerve is 80%. A radial nerve injury above the level of the elbow can result in loss of sensation over the dorsoradial aspect of the hand, inability to extend the metacarpal phalangeal joints of the fingers and thumb, and inability to actively extend the wrist. Active interphalangeal joint extension of the thumb can still be present, owing to the median innervated intrinsic musculature. Treatment of radial nerve palsy resulting from a closed fracture of the distal half of the humerus should include an initial detailed physical examination and baseline electromyogram, followed by observation and a follow-up electromyogram if there is no sign of muscle reinnervation. After an adequate period of observation of generally 2 to 4 months, if there is no sign of improvement, exploration of the radial nerve is appropriate.

If there is radial nerve palsy and the patient has a more distal lesion, such as at the elbow level or the very proximal aspect of the forearm, the extensor carpi ulnaris motor function may be compromised while the extensor carpi radialis muscles may still function, owing to their more proximal level of innervation. This would result in a clinical picture of weak wrist extension and/or extension of the wrist only in a radially deviated direction. In a patient with a high radial nerve palsy, the pronator teres can be used to restore wrist extension, the flexor carpi ulnaris can be transferred to the extensor digitorum communis to restore finger extension, and the palmaris longus can be transferred to the extensor pollicis longus to restore thumb extension.

The posterior interosseous nerve is a branch of the radial nerve. Palsy of the posterior interosseous nerve has been described due to compression resulting from elbow synovitis. Clinically, a patient with such a posterior interosseous nerve palsy may present with the inability to extend only the ulnar digits, with weakness of wrist extension and the inability to ulnarly deviate the wrist in extension. Posterior interosseous nerve lesions can also result from proximal forearm trauma, such as a closed fracture of the proximal ulna with dislocation of the radial head (Monteggia fracture). Treatment of a closed Monteggia fracture generally will include reduction of the fracture and dislocation, and observation of the posterior interosseous nerve palsy.

Compression of the posterior interosseous nerve at the fibrous origin of the supinator muscle can present with many of the same symptoms and clinical picture as lateral epicondylitis.

Recommended Reading

Amillo, S., R. H. Barriose, R. Martinez-Peric, et. al. 1993. Surgical treatment of radial nerve lesions associated with fractures of the humerus. J. Orthop. Trauma, 7:211.

Dawson, D. M., M. Hallett, and L. H. Millender. 1983. Entrapment neuropathies. Boston: Little, Brown.

Green, D. P. 1983. Radial nerve palsy. *In:* Operative hand surgery, 3rd Ed., ed. D. P. Green, 1401. New York: Churchill Livingstone.

Riordan, D. C. 1964. Tendon transfers for nerve paralysis of the hand and wrist. Curr. Prac. Orthop. Surg. 2:17.

Riordan, D. C. 1974. Radial nerve paralysis. Orthop. Clin. North Am. 5:283.

Samardzic, M., D. Grujicic, and Z. B. Milinkovic. 1990. Radial nerve lesions associated with fractures of the humeral shaft. Injury 21:220.

Spinner, M. 1980. Management of nerve compression lesions of the upper extremity. *In:* Management of peripheral nerve problems, ed. G. E. Omer, Jr. and M. Spinner, 569. Philadelphia: W.B. Saunders.

Questions

A. A 20-year-old male has sustained a closed fracture of the midshaft of the right humerus. He is unable to extend the wrist and metacarpophalangeal joint of his right thumb. The likelihood of spontaneous recovery of the radial nerve is:

1. 20%
2. 40%
3. 60%
4. 80%
5. 100%

B. A 25-year-old patient with a humeral shaft fracture and a radial nerve palsy is referred to you 10 weeks after the injury. The fracture was treated with a sugar tong splint and united. The nerve palsy was noted 2 days after the injury. No previous EMGs were obtained. An electromyogram now shows minimal evidence of nerve recovery. The physician should now recommend:

1. Physical therapy and reassessment in 3 months
2. Reevaluation in 1 to 2 months, with a repeat electromyogram
3. Exploration of the nerve now and nerve grafting if necessary
4. Exploration of the nerve and tendon transfers now
5. Tendon transfers

C. A 17-year-old gang member sustains multiple knife wounds to his right arm. He cannot actively extend the metacarpophalangeal joints of his fingers, extend his thumb, or extend his wrist. All other motor function at the elbow, forearm, wrist, and hand is normal. The most likely nerve injury would be a:

1. Partial laceration of the ulnar nerve in the cubital tunnel and complete laceration of the radial nerve deep to the supinator
2. Partial laceration of the median nerve deep to the lacertus fibrosus and partial laceration of the radial nerve deep to the supinator
3. Partial laceration of the median nerve deep to the lacertus fibrosus and complete laceration of the radial nerve deep to the supinator
4. Partial laceration of the radial nerve deep to the supinator
5. Complete laceration of the radial nerve at the level of the intermuscular septum

D. A 22-year-old man who has a synovial sarcoma of the posterior arm undergoes resection of the triceps muscle and a 10-cm segment of the radial nerve. A tumor workup 1 year later revealed no evidence of local tumor recurrence or metastatic spread, and the patient requests treatment to restore function to his wrist, thumb, and fingers. The most appropriate tendon transfers would be:

1. Pronator teres to the extensor carpi radialis brevis, flexor carpi ulnaris to the long finger extensors, and palmaris longus to the extensor pollicis longus
2. Pronator teres to the extensor carpi radialis brevis, flexor carpi ulnaris to the long finger extensors, and flexor carpi radialis to the extensor pollicis longus
3. Brachioradialis to the extensor carpi radialis longus, flexor carpi radialis to the long finger extensors, and extensor indicis proprius to the extensor pollicis longus
4. Brachioradialis to the extensor carpi radialis brevis, flexor carpi ulnaris to the long finger extensors, and extensor indicis proprius to the extensor pollicis longus
5. Flexor carpi radialis to the extensor carpi radialis brevis, extensor indicis proprius to the long finger extensors, and abductor pollicis longus to the extensor pollicis longus

E. A 45-year-old laborer presents with a closed Monteggia fracture of his right forearm. Sensation, circulation, and finger flexion are normal. However, the patient is unable to extend his fingers or thumb. When he extends his wrist, it deviates radially. After reduction of the fracture, your recommendation for treatment of his lack of finger and thumb extension would be:

1. Observation
2. Motor nerve conduction studies of the radial nerve
3. EMGs of the brachioradialis and extensor digitorum communis
4. A dorsal forearm fasciotomy
5. Exploration of the radial nerve

Median Nerve

The most common nerve injury associated with a wrist fracture is a median nerve injury. The median nerve can also be injured in lunate and perilunate fractures and dislocations. Median neuropathy at the level of the carpal tunnel can also result from space-occupying lesions, such as cysts and tumors such as a neurilemoma. The nerve itself may be involved, such as in a neurolipofibroma or neurofibroma. Carpal tunnel syndrome is also seen in association with patients who have been on prolonged renal dialysis.

Carpal tunnel syndrome can result in neurophysiologic changes of the median nerve, including prolongation of motor latency, a decreased thenar compound action potential, prolonged sensory latency, and slowing of the distal conduction velocity. Initial treatment of carpal tunnel syndrome should generally include wrist splinting and nonsteroidal antiinflammatories.

Complications resulting from carpal tunnel surgery can include injury to the motor branch of the median nerve, which would result in compromised function of the superficial head of the flexor pollicis brevis, abductor pollicis brevis, and opponens pollicis. The deep head of the FPB muscle also derives innervation from the deep branch of the ulnar nerve. The palmar cutaneous branch of the median nerve can also be injured, which may result in pain in the wrist and thumb and/or decreased sensation in the thenar area.

Endoscopic release of the carpal tunnel using a single- or a two-portal technique has been reported to result in a quicker return to work on average than that seen following open carpal tunnel release. Endoscopic release of the carpal tunnel has also been associated with complications similar to those reported with an open carpal tunnel release, including ulnar nerve laceration. The most common error committed by an inexperienced surgeon attempting one of his or her first endoscopic carpal tunnel releases using a two-portal technique has been reported to be an incomplete release of the transverse carpal ligament.

The extensor indicis proprius is recommended, when possible, for tendon transfer to restore opposition of the thumb. In a complete high median nerve palsy, the brachioradialis can be transferred to the flexor pollicis longus, and the extensor carpi radialis longus can be transferred to the flexor digitorum profundus of the index and long fingers.

The anterior interosseous nerve is a branch of the median nerve. It has no sensory component and supplies innervation to the flexor pollicis longus muscle, the pronator quadratus, and the flexor digitorum profundus muscle to the index finger and, occasionally, to the long finger profundus muscle as well. Anterior interosseous nerve palsy will result in compromise of precision tip-to-tip pinch between the thumb and index fingers, due to the inability of the patient to flex the DIP joint of the index finger and the IP joint of the thumb. If there is chronic anterior interosseous nerve palsy that is determined to be irreparable and/or there is no hope for reinnervation, function can be improved by arthrodesis of the index finger DIP joint and thumb IP joint.

Recommended Reading

Adams, B. D. 1994. Endoscopic carpal tunnel release. J. Am. Acad. Orthop. Surg. 2:179.

Burkhalter, W. E. 1993. Median nerve palsy. *In:* Operative hand surgery, 3rd Ed., ed. D. P. Green, 1419. New York: Churchill Livingstone.

Dawson, D. M., M. Hallet, and L. H. Millender. 1990. Entrapment neuropathies, 2nd Ed., 111. Boston: Little, Brown.

Dawson, D. M., M. Hallett, and L. H. Millender. 1983. Entrapment neuropathies. Boston: Little, Brown.

Rowland, E. B., and J. M. Kleinert. 1994. Endoscopic carpal tunnel release in cadavera: an investigation of the results of twelve surgeons with this training model. J. Bone Joint Surg. A:266.

Questions

A. The most common nerve injury associated with wrist fractures is to which nerve?

1. Radial
2. Sensory branch of the radial
3. Posterior interosseous
4. Ulnar
5. Median

B. The following neurophysiological changes can all be caused by a carpal tunnel syndrome except:

1. Prolongation of the second digit sensory latency
2. Prolongation of the median motor terminal latency
3. Mild distal conduction slowing in the median nerve
4. Reduction of the thenar compound action potential
5. Fibrillation potential in adductor pollicis

C. During a carpal tunnel release, the motor branch of the median nerve is transected. This complication would most likely result in absence of function in:

1. Superficial and deep head of the flexor pollicis brevis, abductor pollicis brevis, and opponens pollicis
2. Superficial head of the flexor pollicis brevis, adductor pollicis, and opponens pollicis

3. Adductor pollicis and opponens pollicis
4. Deep head of the flexor pollicis brevis, abductor pollicis brevis, and opponens pollicis
5. Superficial and deep heads of the flexor pollicis brevis, adductor pollicis, and opponens pollicis

D. A 23-year-old man presents with a 2-year-old segmental loss of the median nerve in the antecubital region. Which of the following tendon transfers would be most appropriate to reestablish motor function?

1. Flexor carpi radialis to the flexor pollicis longus, brachioradialis to the flexor digitorum profundus of the index and long fingers, and opponensplasty with extensor indicis proprius
2. Flexor digitorum superficialis of the index and long fingers to the flexor digitorum superficialis of the ring and little fingers, extensor carpi radialis longus to the flexor pollicis longus, and opponensplasty with extensor digiti quinti
3. Brachioradialis to the flexor pollicis longus, extensor carpi radialis longus to the flexor digitorum profundus of the index and long fingers, and opponensplasty with extensor indicis proprius
4. Brachioradialis to the flexor pollicis longus, extensor carpi radialis longus to the flexor digitorum profundus of the index and long fingers, and opponensplasty with flexor digitorum superficialis of the long finger
5. Brachioradialis to the flexor pollicis longus, extensor carpi radialis longus to the flexor digitorum profundus of the index and long fingers, and an opponensplasty with flexor digitorum superficialis of the ring finger

E. A 48-year-old roofer slipped while climbing down a ladder, but caught himself by holding onto a ladder rung with his right hand. For 3 weeks after the injury, he had deep, aching pain and swelling of the entire upper extremity. Most of his symptoms have gradually resolved. Eight weeks after the injury, however, he complains of persistent weakness of the thumb. Physical examination reveals that he is unable to actively flex the interphalangeal joint of the thumb or the distal interphalangeal joint of the index finger. There is no apparent sensory or reflex deficit, and the remainder of the upper extremity examination is normal. The diagnosis most likely is:

1. Injury to the anterior interosseous nerve
2. Injury to the medial cord of the brachial plexus
3. Partial lower trunk brachial plexus palsy
4. Anomalous interconnection between the flexor pollicis longus and the index flexor digitorum profundus tendons
5. Rupture of the musculotendinous junctions of the flexor pollicis longus and flexor digitorum profundus to the index finger

F. Which of the following muscles are affected in an anterior interosseous nerve syndrome?

1. Flexor pollicis longus, index flexor digitorum profundus, pronator quadratus
2. Index flexor digitorum superficialis, flexor pollicis brevis
3. Abductor pollicis brevis, opponens pollicis, pronator quadratus
4. Pronator teres, adductor pollicis
5. Long and small finger flexor digitorum superficialis

G. A 28-year-old, right-handed carpenter had an open reduction and plate fixation of midshaft left radius and ulna fractures over 2 years ago. The fractures have healed, but he still has problems holding a nail between his index finger and thumb. Physical examination reveals weakness of thumb to index tip pinch. The most appropriate treatment for this patient is:

1. Continued observation
2. Exploration and repair of the involved nerve
3. Tenolysis of the involved tendons
4. Muscle-strengthening exercises
5. Arthrodesis of the index distal interphalangeal joint and thumb interphalangeal joints

Musculocutaneous Nerve

The musculocutaneous nerve can be injured during anterior shoulder surgery around the coracoid process. Injury to the musculocutaneous nerve at the level of the shoulder can result in weakened shoulder adduction, elbow flexion, and forearm supination. Sensory changes, including dysesthesias in the anterolateral aspect of the elbow and forearm, can also occur. Compression of the musculocutaneous nerve by the biceps aponeurosis can result in dysesthesia in the anterolateral aspect of the elbow and forearm, which can be accentuated by pronation and supination of the forearm.

Recommended Reading

Dawson, D. M., M. Hallett, and L. H. Millender. 1983. Entrapment neuropathies. Boston: Little, Brown.

Questions

A. A 29-year-old male complains of burning dysesthesia in the anterolateral elbow and forearm accentuated by pronation and supination of the forearm. What peripheral nerve is involved?

1. Radial
2. Musculocutaneous
3. Median
4. Antebrachial cutaneous
5. Lateral cutaneous

8 The Thumb

A complete tear of the ulnar collateral ligament of the thumb metacarpal phalangeal joint can be a disabling injury. This injury has been called a "gamekeeper's thumb." It has also been called a "skier's thumb." However, it can result from any activity or injury that results in hyperabduction of the thumb. It is important to discern whether there is an avulsion fracture associated with the ligament injury and whether or not the rupture is complete. If there is no fracture component to the injury and it is a complete ligament tear, there is a significant chance that the ligament would have avulsed off the base of the proximal phalanx and lies reflected back on itself with the adductor aponeurosis and extensor hood of the thumb interposed between the ligament and its normal area of attachment. This type of pathoanatomy was described by Stener and will not heal if treated nonsurgically (Fig. 8–1). Stress testing in at least 30° of flexion is important to assess whether the disruption is complete. Complete disruption of the ulnar collateral ligament will result in greater than 40° of instability with radially directed stress on the proximal phalanx of the thumb when the MCP joint is in 30° of flexion. Complete disruption of the ulnar collateral ligament is associated with some degree of disruption of the capsule of the MCP joint. If the disruption is determined to be complete and has no avulsion fracture component, the injury should be surgically explored and the ligament repaired.

Another injury that can occur to the thumb is the so-called Bennett's fracture, in which there is an oblique, intraarticular fracture of the base of the first metacarpal. The first metacarpal dislocates dorsally and proximally, due primarily to the action of the abductor pollicis longus (Fig. 8–2).

The first carpal metacarpal joint is a common location for degenerative arthritis to occur, particularly in women in their 60s and 70s. It is also important to assess the scaphotrapeziotrapezoid joints, because the pattern of arthritis can be a pantrapezial distribution. At one time, the treatment preference was either a silastic implant arthroplasty for the

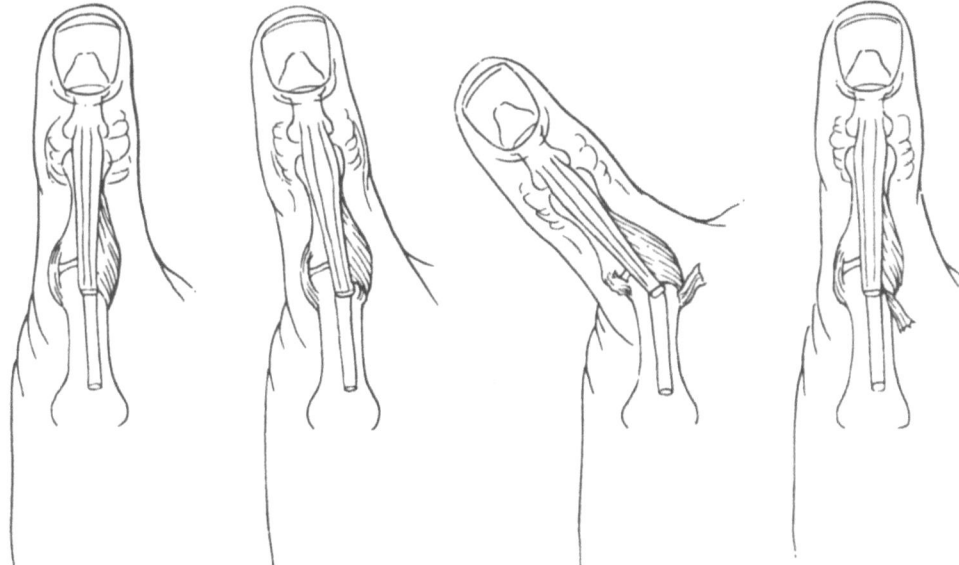

Fig. 8-1. From left to right, the sequence of hyperabduction of the thumb MP joint in which the ulnar collateral ligament can be avulsed off the proximal ulnar base of the thumb proximal phalanx; and, as the extensor mechanism of the thumb relocates, the ulnar collateral ligament can fold back on itself. This type of pathoanatomy was described by Stener and is sometimes called a Stener lesion.

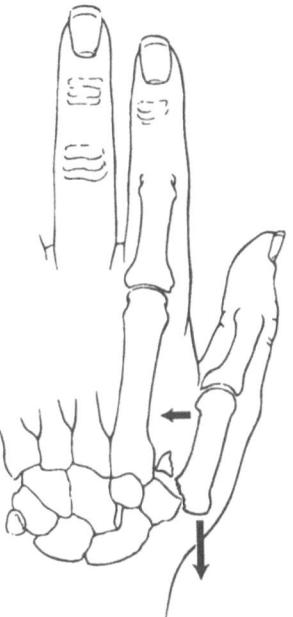

Fig. 8-2. A Bennett's fracture in which the volar base of the thumb metacarpal remains in a reduced posture. The remainder of the first metacarpal fractures away from it and dislocates in a proximal direction from the pull of the abductor pollicis longus tendon, and the thumb assumes a somewhat adducted posture.

CMC joint if the arthritis was localized to this area, or resection of the trapezium with a trapezial silastic implant if the arthritis was pantrapezial. Due to the problems with silastic synovitis, however, the current treatment recommendation is a soft tissue interpositional arthroplasty. If there is sufficient hyperextension instability of the MP joint, the MP joint should be stabilized. If there is IP joint arthritis, fusion of the IP joint generally results in satisfactory results. The preferred position of IP joint fusion is 10° of flexion, neutral abduction/adduction, and 5° of pronation. If a patient presents who has been treated with a silastic implant and has developed silicone synovitis, management should be excision of the silastic implant.

A boutonniere deformity of the thumb includes flexion at the metacarpal phalangeal joint and hyperextension at the IP joint of the thumb. This thumb deformity pattern is most commonly the result of pathology primarily at the metacarpal phalangeal joint of the thumb (Fig. 8–3). A swan neck deformity of the thumb includes subluxation of the base of the thumb metacarpal in relation to the trapezium, an adducted posture of the thumb metacarpal, with hyperextension of the metacarpal phalangeal joint of the thumb and flexion of the interphalangeal joint of the thumb. This deformity develops primarily at the carpal metacarpal joint with the metacarpal phalangeal joint and interphalangeal joint postures developing secondarily (Fig. 8–4).

Thumb opposition is an important function of the thumb. If absent, the extensor indicis proprius or, alternatively, flexor digitorum sublimis, usually of the ring finger, can be used for tendon transfers to restore thumb opposition. A majority of congenital trigger digits involve the thumb alone and may be associated with permanent interphalangeal joint flexion contracture. If the congenital trigger thumb does not resolve spontaneously, it will respond immediately to release of the A-1 pulley. Thumb-in-palm deformity in a patient with cerebral palsy is best surgically managed by metacarpophalangeal joint arthrodesis, tendon transfer, and release of the first dorsal interosseous and adductor muscles. The thumb is one of the more commonly involved digits with regard to polydactyly (Fig. 8–5). Treatment of polydactyly involving the thumb generally includes utilization of components from each thumb to reconstruct as anatomically and functionally complete a thumb as possible. Simple amputation of one of the thumbs and failure to adequately reconstruct the remaining digit can result in subsequent instability and/or deformity. Undergrowth or hypoplasia of the thumb can also occur. A floating thumb, or so-called *pouce flottant*, should be treated with amputation of the thumb and pollicization of the index finger (Fig. 8–6). The ability of these children, who have had a pollicization of the index finger, to handle large objects shows the most improvement.

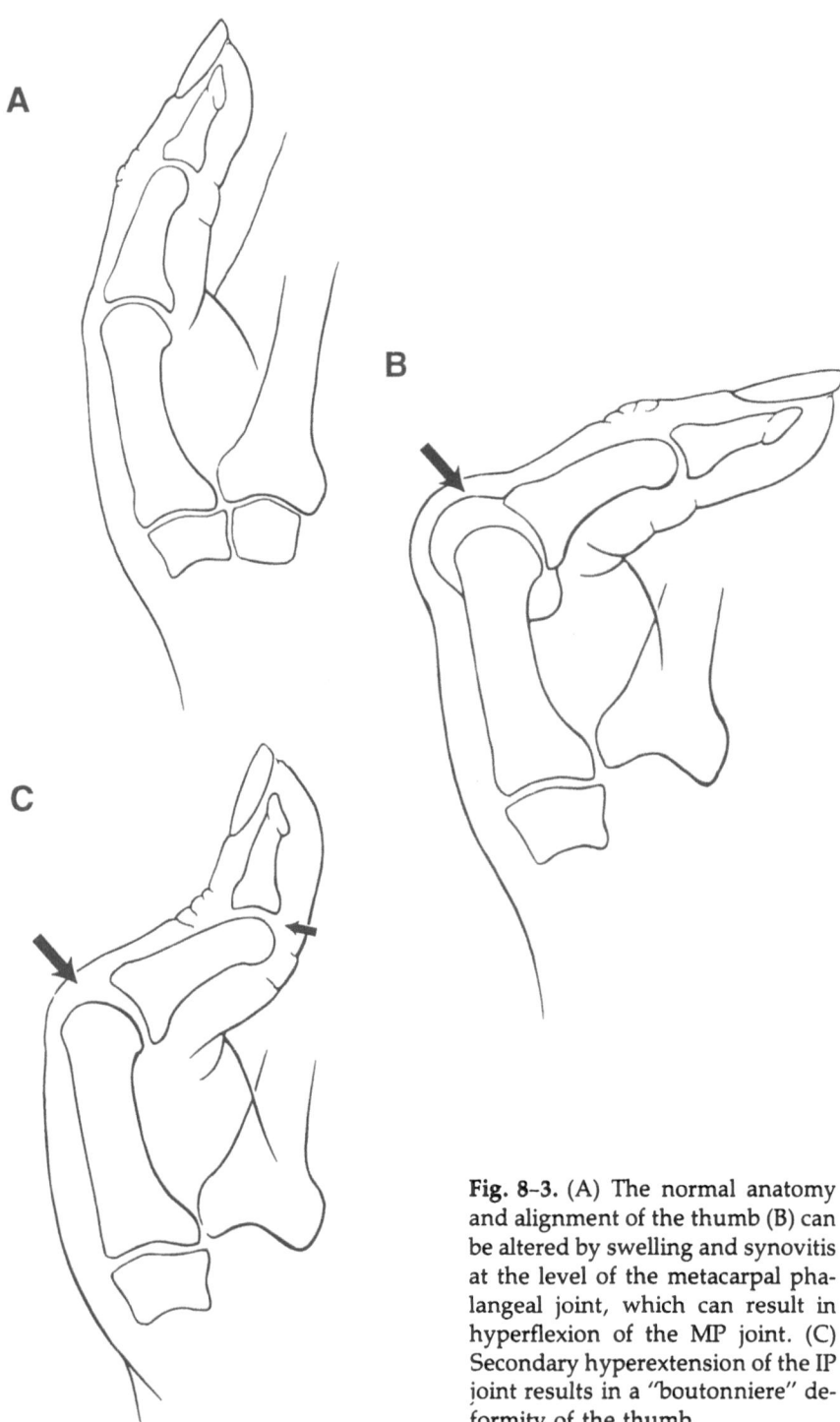

A

B

C

Fig. 8-3. (A) The normal anatomy and alignment of the thumb (B) can be altered by swelling and synovitis at the level of the metacarpal phalangeal joint, which can result in hyperflexion of the MP joint. (C) Secondary hyperextension of the IP joint results in a "boutonniere" deformity of the thumb.

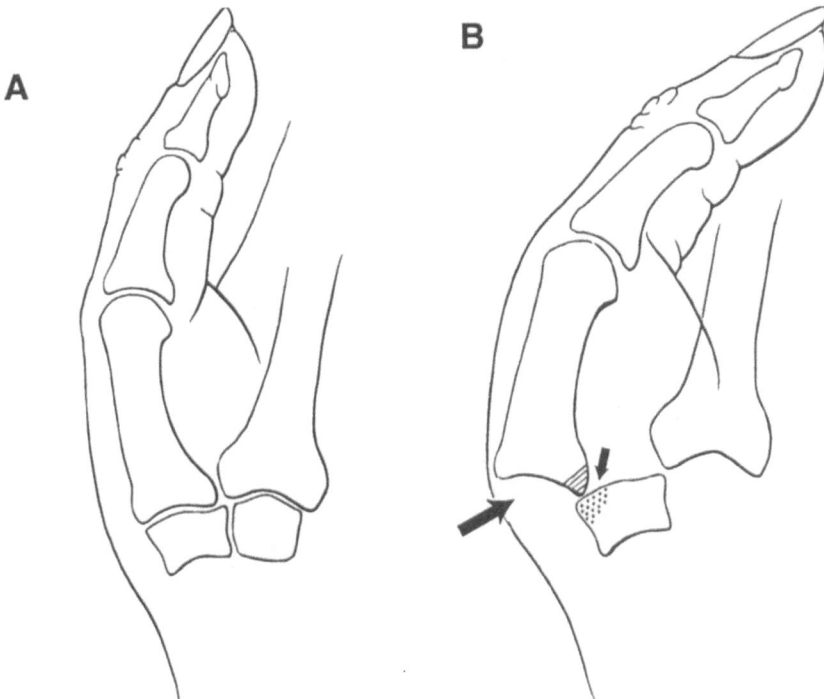

Fig. 8-4. (A) The normal anatomy and alignment of the thumb can also be altered, (B) by laxity and subluxation of the first metacarpal in relation to the trapezium, resulting in incongruous loading of that joint (lined and dotted areas).

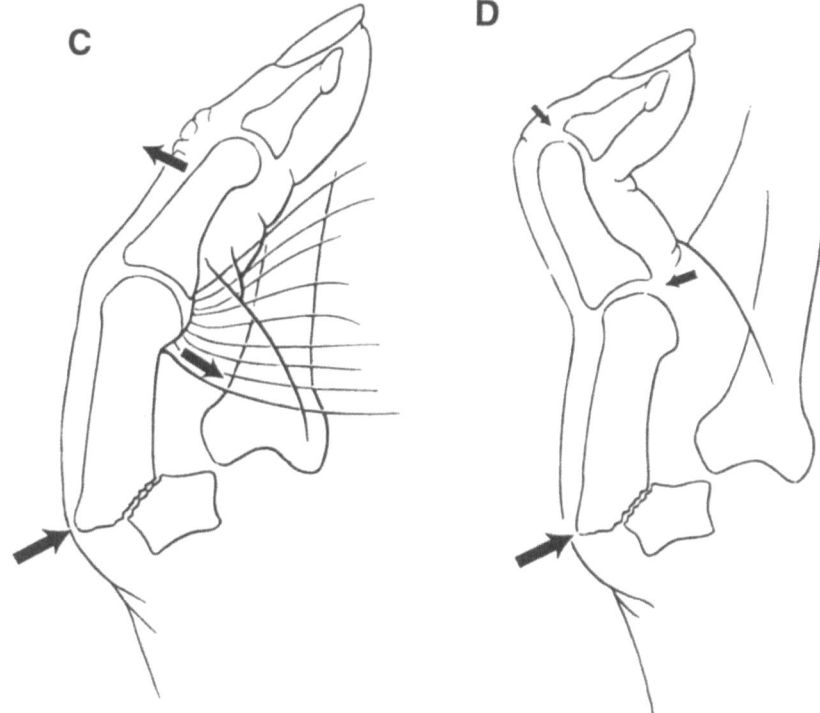

Fig. 8-4. (C) Secondary joint space changes and erosion can result in prominence at the base of the first metacarpal with the first metacarpal in an adducted posture. (D) There then develops a secondary stretching of the volar plate at the MP joint with hyperextension of the thumb MP joint, and subsequent compensatory hyperflexion of the IP joint of the thumb to accomplish pinching and grasping. This subsequent deformity is called a swan neck deformity of the thumb.

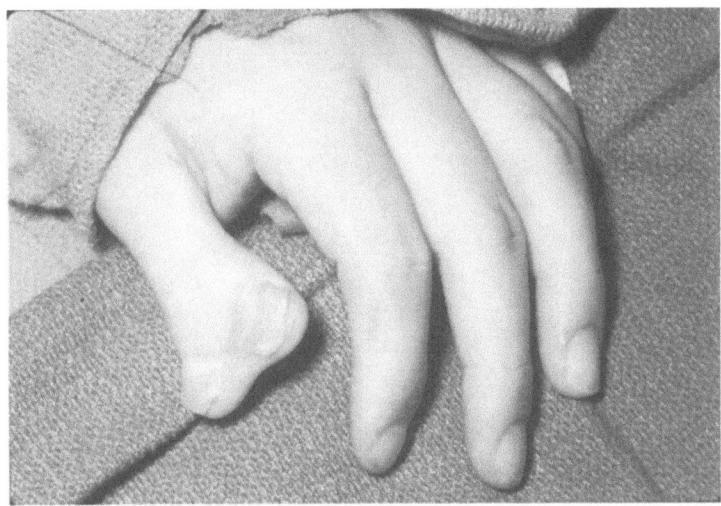

Fig. 8-5. A clinical photograph of a type I bifid thumb.

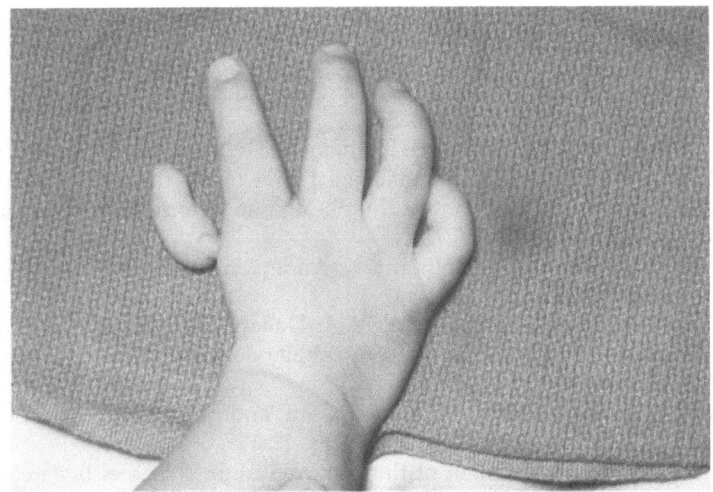

a

Fig. 8-6. (a) Clinical photograph of a patient with the so-called *pouce flottant* or floating thumb.

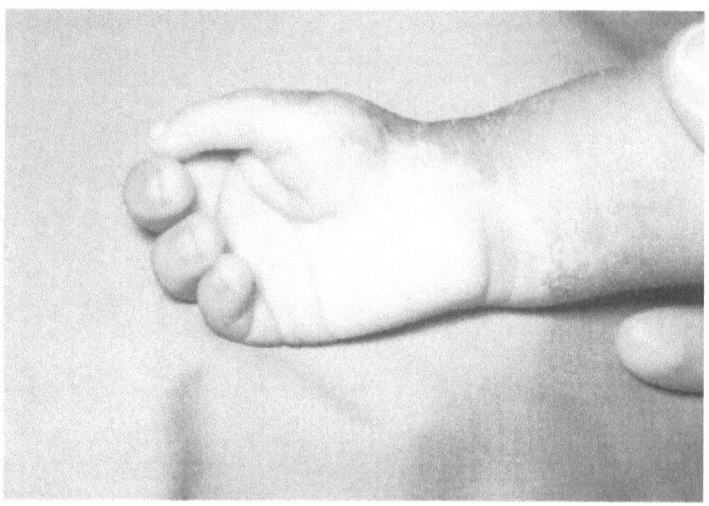

b

Fig. 8-6. (b) A photograph of the same hand following amputation of the floating thumb and pollicization of the index finger.

Recommended Reading

Cooney, W. P., D. Arnold, and J. Grace. 1990. Collateral ligament injury of the thumb. Adv. Orthop. Surg. 13:235.

Goldner, J. L., A. L. Koman, R. Gelberman, S. Levin, and R. D. Goldner. 1990. Arthrodesis of the metacarpophalangeal joint of the thumb in children and adults. Adjunctive treatment of thumb-in-palm deformity in cerebral palsy. Clin. Orthop. Rel. Res. 253:75.

Kjaer-Petersen, K., O. Langhoff, and K. Andersen. 1990. Bennett's fracture. J. Hand Surg. 15:58.

Manske, P. R., M. D. Rotman, and L. A. Dailey. 1992. Long term functional results after pollicization for the congenitally deficient thumb. J. Hand Surg. 17A:1064.

Nalebuff, E. A. 1968. Diagnosis, classification, and management of rheumatoid thumb deformities. Bull. Hosp. Joint Dis. 29:119.

Stener, B. 1962. Displacement of the ruptured ulnar collateral ligament of the metacarpal phalangeal joint of the thumb: a clinical and anatomical study. J. Bone Joint Surg. 44B:869.

Questions

A. A 20-year-old woman injures the metacarpophalangeal joint of her thumb while skiing. Examination reveals well-localized tenderness along the ulnar aspect of the metacarpophalangeal joint. With the metacarpophalangeal joint in full extension, radially directed stress provides less than 5° of angulation. With the metacarpophalangeal joint held in flexion, 45° of angulation occurs. Radiographs are normal. Treatment should consist of:

1. A thumb splint and reassessment in 3 weeks
2. A short arm thumb spica cast for 6 weeks
3. Repair of the volar plate
4. Repair of the ulnar collateral ligament and capsule
5. Adductor pollicis advancement on the middle phalanx

B. The dislocation of the first metacarpal in a Bennett's fracture-dislocation of the thumb is caused primarily by the force of the:

1. Opponens pollicis
2. Adductor pollicis
3. Flexor pollicis longus
4. Flexor pollicis brevis
5. Abductor pollicis longus

C. Congenital trigger thumb:

1. Is caused by an enlarged sesamoid bone
2. Is caused by a constriction of the flexor pollicis longus at the oblique ligament
3. May be associated with permanent interphalangeal joint flexion contracture
4. Is associated with congenital absence of the extensor pollicis longus
5. Is associated with congenital contracture of the flexor pollicis longus

9 Infections

It is important to know the anatomy of the various spaces in the hand (Fig. 9-1), and the location and extent of the various flexor tendon sheaths (Fig. 9-2). Infectious processes follow anatomic plains and spaces when they spread. A purulent flexor tenosynovitis of the third, fourth, and fifth fingers that extends proximally can involve the mid-palmar space. Involvement of the index finger and thumb with proximal extension would involve the thenar space. The hypothenar space contains the hypothenar muscles and rarely is involved with a deep space infection. Improper treatment, as well as delay in beginning treatment of infections of the hand, can result in disastrous outcomes. Human bites of the hand can result in severe infections. A common mechanism of injury is when one individual strikes another person in the mouth with a clenched fist and sustains a puncture wound, usually into the knuckle, from a tooth of the individual that was struck. One organism commonly associated with human bites is *Eikenella corrodens*, a microaerophilic, anaerobic, gram-negative rod. Penicillin and ampicillin are effective against *Eikenella*. Although *Eikenella corrodens* is commonly associated with human bites, the most common infecting organism is still *Staphylococcus aureus*. Appropriate treatment of this so-called "fight bite" should include irrigation and debridement, and administration of appropriate antibiotic coverage. Exploration of the wound should include not only debridement of the wound, but also irrigation and debridement of the metacarpal phalangeal joint if the fight bite wound overlies the MCP joint. The wound should be left open and the digit should be splinted. The most frequent long-term complication of this injury is osteomyelitis and pyarthrosis. Dog and cat bites of the hand can also result in severe infections. The organism often associated with domestic animal bites is *Pasturella multocida*, a small, gram-negative coccus. The antibiotic of choice for this organism is penicillin.

An infection of the flexor tendon sheath can result in severe disability. Infection within the flexor tendon sheath can destroy the gliding mechanism and quickly create adhesions, resulting in limitation of

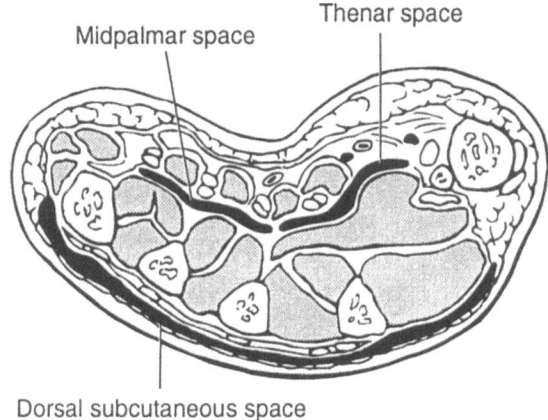

Fig. 9-1. An illustration demonstrating the various spaces in a cross section of the hand.

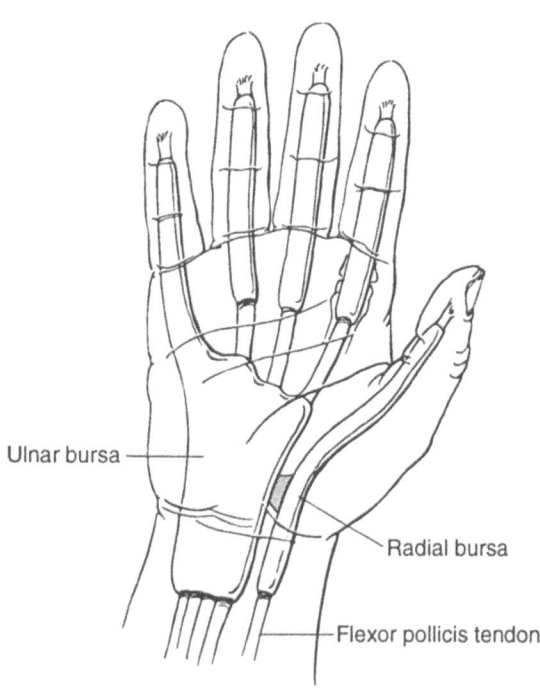

Fig. 9-2. An illustration showing the flexor tendon sheaths of the hand. There can be an intercommunication (shaded area) between the flexor pollicis longus tendon sheath and the midpalmar flexor tendon sheath.

tendon function and loss of motion. The vincula blood supply of the flexor tendons can be destroyed from a flexor tendon sheath infection and can result in tendon necrosis. The most common pathogen, again, is *Staphylococcus aureus*. Dr Alan B. Kanavel described what he felt were the four classic findings of infected flexor tenosynovitis: (1) a flexed position of the finger; (2) symmetric or fusiform swelling of the finger; (3) excessive tenderness over the course of the flexor tendon sheath; and (4) Severe pain on passive extension of the finger. Pain on passive extension of the finger is the most valuable, and may be the only finding present in very early septic flexor tenosynovitis. There are a variety of operative methods described to treat septic flexor tenosynovitis. All of the methods require adequate irrigation and debridement of the flexor tendon sheath, whether through surgical exposure of the entire sheath with debridement of the flexor tendon sheath and salvage of the annular pulleys, or through limited incisions and catheter irrigation.

There are several types of mycobacteria that have been reported to cause infections in the hand. The most common is *Mycobacterium marinum*. A patient with an atypical mycobacterial infection often has a history of a penetrating wound sustained in a marine environment. Alternatively, the source of the organism can be from warm, freshwater lakes or tropical aquariums. For appropriate identification, the cultures must be incubated at 30° to 32°C, rather than the usual culture temperature of 37°C. Microscopically, the specimens will show noncaseating granulomas and acid-fast bacilli. Optimal treatment typically includes a combination of surgical debridement and antituberculous medication, which may include Ethambutol and Rifampin for at least 6 to 9 months.

Other infections can include gonococcal infections in the joints or flexor tendon sheaths of the hand. These usually respond well to intravenous penicillin. Tuberculosis, although not common, can also result in hand infections and can present with a similar clinical picture to that of a mycobacterial infection. Tuberculosis dactylitis can cause enlarged fingers which, on radiograph, show a subperiosteal reaction. Leprosy *M lepraemurium*, as with atypical mycobacterial infections, demonstrates a preference for the cooler areas of the body, such as the extremities. Leprosy commonly affects the hands, often producing a neuropathy that most commonly involves the ulnar nerve in the hand.

Painful infections of the digits may result from the herpes simplex virus. Unnecessary surgical intervention may result in increased morbidity of this otherwise essentially benign and self-limiting process. There is an apparently high incidence of herpes simplex virus infections of the digits in medical and dental personnel. Herpes infection of the hand was originally described in 1909. Stern et al coined the phrase "herpetic whitlow" in 1959. Patients with herpetic whitlow should be restricted from patient contact, and the lesion, which typically will be erythematous, tender to palpation, and have several small vesicles containing clear fluid, should simply be observed.

Various anaerobic and aerobic organisms can cause gas-producing infections in the hand and forearm. Classic gas gangrene results from a *Clostridium* infection. Clostridial organisms are a gram-positive rod. The history of a patient with a clostridial infection will often include a wound, sometimes just a small puncture wound, that is contaminated by dirt. These infections can rapidly become severe and pose a threat to both life and limb if not treated appropriately and expediently. These infections often are associated with severe pain, tense skin with other areas of hemorrhagic bulli, and compromised muscle. A serosanguineous discharge can also be evident from any wounds. Treatment should include adequate debridement of any necrotic tissue and appropriate antibiotic therapy, such as penicillin, metronidazole (Flagyl), or clindamycin. At times, hyperbaric oxygen therapy can be added to the treatment regimen.

Recommended Reading

Gill, J. M., J. Arlette, and K. Buchan. 1988. Herpes simplex virus infection of the hand. A profile of 79 cases. Am. J. Med. 84:89.

Lacy, J. N., S. F. Viegas, J. H. Calhoun, and J. T. Mader. 1989. *Mycobacterium marinum* flexor tenosynovitis. Clin. Orthop. Rel. Res. 238:288.

Neviaser, R. J. 1993. Infections. *In:* Operative hand surgery, 3rd Ed., ed. D. P. Green, 1021.

Stern, H., S. D. Elek, D. M. Millar, and H. F. Anderson. 1959. Herpetic whitlow: a form of cross-infection in hospitals. Lancet 11:871.

Questions

A. A 23-year-old man presents to the Emergency Room with a 3-day history of swelling, pain, tenderness, and erythema over the dorsum of the metacarpophalangeal joint of his right index finger. Examination of the hand reveals a small, irregular laceration over the metacarpal head, with some erythema surrounding the wound. Radiographs are normal. The recommended treatment should be:

1. Irrigation of the wound, dressing changes, and splinting of the hand
2. Splinting of the hand and oral antibiotics
3. Splinting of the hand and intravenous antibiotics
4. Debridement of the wound and intravenous antibiotics
5. Debridement of the metacarpophalangeal joint and intravenous antibiotics

B. A 21-year-old man has pain and swelling of the right hand third metacarpal-phalangeal joint 18 hours after injuring it in a fist fight. Examination of the hand reveals a healing wound over the metacarpal head and erythema surrounding the wound. The most appropriate treatment would be:

1. Rest, soaks, and elevation
2. Debridement, wound closure, and antibiotics
3. Aspiration and cultures
4. Immobilization and IV antibiotics
5. Debridement, leave the wound open, and antibiotics

C. A 27-year-old woman is bitten by her cat in the index finger. Ten days later, she presents with an infected flexor tendon sheath of the index finger. The wound is incised and drained; cultures grow *Pasteurella multocida*. The most appropriate antibiotic treatment for this organism is:

1. Keflin
2. Penicillin G
3. Gentamicin
4. Vancomycin
5. Rifampin

D. A 32-year-old woman has pain and swelling of her ring finger 48 hours after sustaining a puncture wound in the PIP joint flexion crease. Physical examination of the hand reveals fusiform swelling of the finger, tenderness to palpation along the palmar surface of the finger extending to the distal palmar crease, extreme pain with passive extension of the finger, and limited active flexion due to pain. The physician should recommend:

1. Elevation, splinting, oral antibiotics, and observation
2. Tendon sheath aspiration, IV antibiotics, and splinting
3. Flexor tenosynovectomy and IV antibiotics
4. Incision, drainage, and irrigation of the flexor tendon sheath through a limited palmar and a distal finger incision, and IV antibiotics
5. Incision, drainage, and irrigation of the flexor tendon sheath through separate digital, palmar, and wrist incisions, and IV antibiotics

E. A 35-year-old man presents 10 weeks after he had lacerated his thumb while fishing. Examination reveals pain, swelling, and erythema of his thumb and thenar area. Material obtained during surgical debridement is sent for culture. What one laboratory technique will increase the likelihood that the pathogen will be identified?

1. Culturing the specimen at 30°C (86°F)
2. Culturing the specimen at 38°C (100.4°F)
3. Culturing the specimen under anaerobic conditions

4. Culturing the specimen on a Thayer Martin media
5. Use of a potassium hydroxide preparation

F. A 32-year-old dentist has pain and swelling over the pulp of his right thumb. Examination reveals that the pulp is erythematous, tender, and has several small vesicles containing clear fluid. The dentist denies any history of trauma or injury to the thumb. The physician should recommend avoiding contact with patients and:

1. Observation
2. Oral antibiotics for 10 to 14 days
3. Splinting, IV antibiotics, and observation
4. Incision and drainage of the vesicles
5. Incision and drainage of the digital pulp

G. 48-year-old man sustained multiple lacerations and puncture wounds in his right forearm when he fell onto his rake while gardening. The wounds were irrigated and closed primarily, and the patient was given a 3-day course of an oral cephalosporin. He presents 5 days after the injury. His oral temperature is 102°F, his pulse is 120/min, his blood pressure is 90/40 mm Hg, and he is diaphoretic. He has severe pain in the forearm, the skin is tense with areas of hemorrhagic bullae, and there is dusky muscle bulging from the lacerations. He also has a serosanguineous discharge from the wounds. A Gram's stain of the discharge reveals a few white cells and scattered, large gram-positive bacilli. Radiographs of the patient's forearm show interstitial gas. The physician should first:

1. Start a third-generation cephalosporin and measure forearm compartment pressures
2. Open all incision sites, irrigate thoroughly, pack the wounds open, and start IV penicillin
3. Open all incision sites, irrigate thoroughly, pack the wounds open, and start IV cephalosporin, gentamicin, and penicillin
4. Debride the necrotic muscle and start a third-generation cephalosporin
5. Debride the necrotic muscle and start IV penicillin and hyperbaric oxygen

H. A 55-year-old man with diabetes has increasing pain, tenderness, and swelling of the palm. Examination reveals tenderness over the palm and thenar eminence. The patient has pain with any attempt to actively flex the thumb and index finger. This patient probably has a:

1. Felon
2. Midpalmar space infection
3. Thenar space infection
4. Flexor tendon sheath infection of the thumb
5. Flexor tendon sheath infection of the index finger

10 Arthritis

Rheumatoid arthritis is a chronic, systemic, autoimmune, inflammatory disease that affects joints and periarticular tissues. Rheumatoid arthritis can cause a number of different deformities and functional impairment in the hand.

The metacarpal phalangeal joints of the fingers are common sites for rheumatoid involvement and cause MP joint synovitis, which distends and stretches the joint capsule and attenuates the collateral ligaments (Figs. 10-1 and 10-2). This results in palmar subluxation of the proximal phalanx and intrinsic muscle tightness. Both add to the tendency for the fingers to posture in a swan neck deformity and/or to develop ulnar drift of the digits. If there is Hyperextension of the proximal interphalangeal joint with limitation of proximal interphalangeal flexion with the metacarpal phalangeal joint in any position dorsal subluxation and contracture of the lateral bands of the extensor hood will be present. Rheumatoid arthritis boutonniere deformities, where the PIP joint is in flexion with DIP joint hyperextension, will typically occur as a result of PIP joint synovitis, which causes elongation and/or rupture of the central slip and volar subluxation of the lateral bands to a position palmar to the PIP joint axis of rotation. Pain-limited motion and radiographic evidence of joint destruction in the DIP joints are generally treated by arthrodesing the DIP joint. Similar changes at the PIP joint level are also treated with arthrodesis in the index and little fingers. If there is PIP joint involvement in the long or ring fingers, a PIP joint arthroplasty can be an alternative to arthrodesis.

A swan neck deformity of the thumb generally develops from laxity and degenerative changes in the carpal metacarpal joint with dorsal subluxation of the metacarpal in relation to the trapezium. Secondary changes, due to the imbalance caused by dorsal subluxation of the proximal portion of the thumb metacarpal and an adducted posture of the first metacarpal, will result in hyperextension of the metacarpal phalangeal joint of the thumb and hyperflexion of the interphalangeal joint of the thumb. A boutonniere deformity of the thumb includes

93

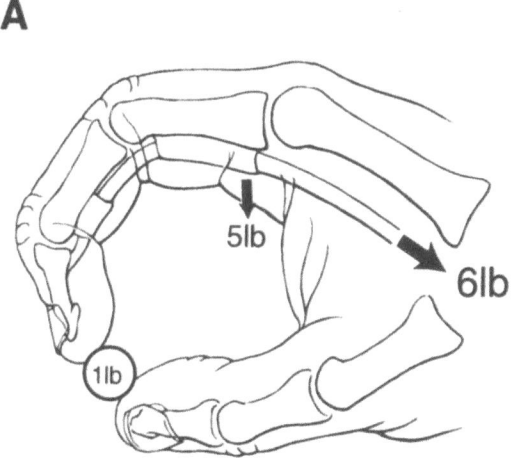

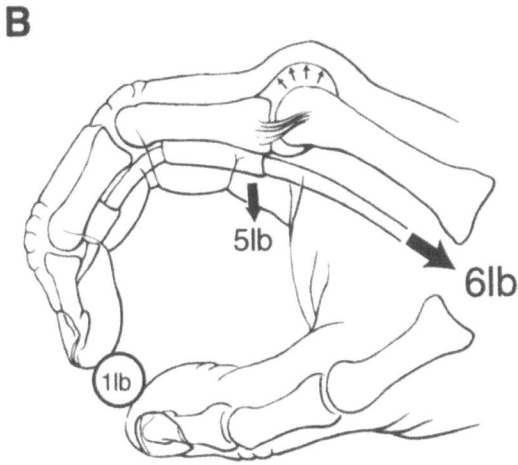

Fig. 10-1. A series of illustrations showing the progression (A) from a normal joint alignment to (B) MP joint synovitis and attenuation of the collateral ligaments and capsule, which allows volar subluxation of the proximal phalanx in relation to the metacarpal head, due to the normal biomechanic forces in the hand and digits.

C

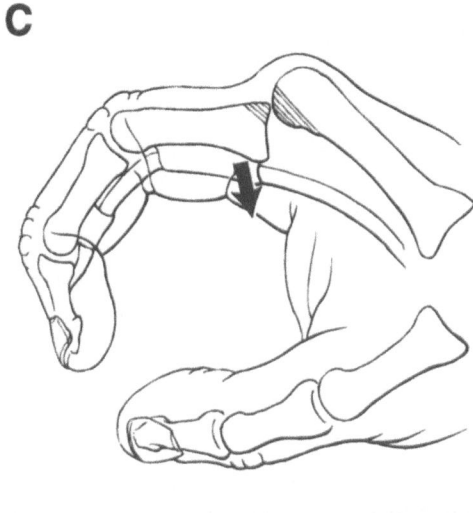

D

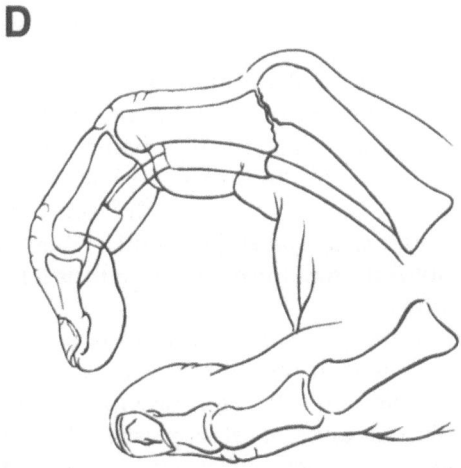

Fig. 10-1. (cont'd) (C) The resulting incongruous articulation results in wear of the dorsal base of the proximal phalanx and the volar aspect of the metacarpal head, resulting (D) in the typical appearance of an end-stage deformity of the MP joint in a patient with rheumatoid arthritis.

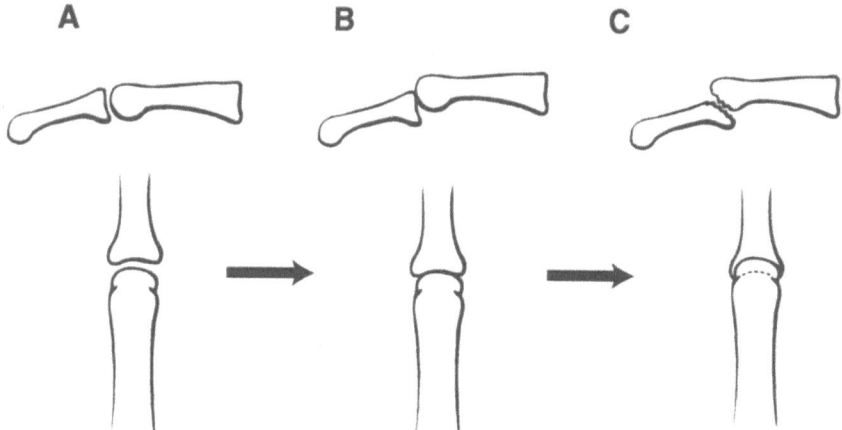

Fig. 10-2. This series shows the same sequence as in Figure 10-1, which illustrates the change in the metacarpophalangeal joint space seen on radiographs (A) in a normal joint, (B) in a joint with synovitis and subluxation of the MP joint, and (C) in a joint with subluxation and joint erosion showing the typical overlap of the base of the proximal phalanx on the metacarpal head.

flexion of the metacarpal phalangeal joint and hyperextension of the interphalangeal joint of the thumb. Treatment can include fusion of the interphalangeal joint and transfer and advancement of the extensor pollicis longus to the base of the proximal phalanx of the thumb. The primary involvement in a boutonniere deformity of the thumb is typically at the metacarpal phalangeal joint, where synovitis allows attenuation and subluxation of the extensor pollicis longus and extensor pollicis brevis tendons.

The carpal metacarpal joint of the thumb is a common location of osteoarthritic involvement in the thumb, occurring most commonly in women in their 60s and 70s. Although previous treatment recommendations included silicone implant arthroplasties, because of silicone synovitis this treatment has fallen out of favor, and a soft tissue interposition arthroplasty is now generally the preferred treatment. Close evaluation should always be made of the scaphoid-trapezium-trapezoid joint, because the degenerative changes may be pantrapezial, in which case excision of the trapezium and a soft tissue interposition and ligament suspension plasty of the first metacarpal should be performed. If any excessive hyperextension instability of the MP joint exists, this should also be corrected. A patient with rheumatoid arthritis who has decreasing, active flexion of the digits while maintaining full passive range of motion should be assessed for flexor tenosynovitis. If the patient does not respond to medical management, a flexor tenosynovectomy is appropriate management. A patient with significant flexor tenosynovitis that is uncontrolled may rupture one or more flexor tendons.

The extensor tendons are much more likely than the flexor tendons to rupture in a patient with rheumatoid arthritis. If significant dorsal tenosynovitis persists, despite 6 months of adequate and appropriate medical management, a dorsal tenosynovectomy is the treatment of choice and an effective means of preventing extensor tendon rupture. If left untreated, a rupture of the extensor digitorum communis tendons, usually starting with the tendons to the most ulnar digits, may occur. The most common site for a rupture of the extensor digitorum communis tendons is at the distal border of the extensor retinaculum at the level of the distal ulna head. Clinical examination of a patient in whom there is a question of extensor tendon rupture should include passive flexion and extension of the wrist. If the extensor tendons are intact, passive flexion of the wrist should result in a relative extension posturing of the fingers. This is the so-called passive tenodesis effect. It is important to differentiate extensor tendon ruptures from posterior interosseous nerve palsy, extensor mechanism subluxation, and MP joint dislocation. Function of the extensor digitorum quinti is tested by holding the index, long, and ring fingers in flexion to eliminate the function of the extensor digitorum communis tendons and having the patient actively extend the small finger. Multiple tendon ruptures can be treated by bridge grafting, adjacent tendon suture repair, or tendon transfer. If the distal ulna is arthritic and a source of attritional wear of the tendons, the distal ulna should be resected. The extensor indicis proprius tendon is a good donor for tendon transfer to restore finger extension or thumb extension when the extensor pollicis longus tendon has ruptured.

Evaluation of intrinsic tightness can be accomplished by assessing the resistance to passive flexion of the PIP joint with the metacarpal phalangeal joint held extended and aligned with the metacarpal of that finger, and then retested with the MP joint flexed. If there is more resistance to passive PIP joint flexion and more limited flexion of the PIP joint with the MP joint extended than flexed, there is intrinsic tightness.

Synovitis of the distal radioulnar joint will lead to palmar subluxation of the radius and carpus, which is conventionally called dorsal subluxation or dislocation of the ulna. This deformity can be a contributing factor to extensor tendon rupture in rheumatoid arthritis. A distal ulna resection, synovectomy, and appropriate tendon repairs or transfers are appropriate in the treatment of this condition. Ulnar neuropathy at Guyon's canal may be found in association with this pathology. If there is significant destruction of the proximal and midcarpal joints, wrist fusion is an acceptable treatment with predictable results. When assessing a patient with rheumatoid arthritis, the entire extremity should be assessed. The elbow may also be involved. Depending on the extent of joint involvement and destruction, the patient's symptoms and function may be improved by a synovectomy, interposition fascial arthroplasty, or total elbow replacement.

Gout can cause one of the two types of crystal-induced arthritis. The other type of crystal-induced arthritis is pseudogout. Gout can cause the deposition in tissue of monosodium urate crystals, resulting from sustained hyperuricemia. Roentgenographic findings of patients with gouty arthritis usually include sharply marginated periarticular bony defects. The association of an erosive bone lesion adjacent to a radio-dense soft tissue mass, due to calcification of the tophus, is pathognomonic of gout. Treatment of acute gout can be addressed with indomethicin or colchicine, while the prevention of recurrent gouty attacks is generally treated with allopurinol.

Scleroderma, or systemic sclerosis, is a multisystem disease which often affects the hands. Patients with scleroderma often have Raynaud's phenomenon, with cold intolerance. Secretan's disease (peritendinous fibrosis) of the dorsum of the hand has been reported in association with a number of factors including self-mutilation, compensatable work-related injuries, and psychosis, neurosis, and suicidal tendency. Reiter's syndrome is defined as the association of nonbacterial urethritis, arthritis, and conjunctivitis. Reiter's syndrome rarely involves the hand and more commonly involves the knees ankles and feet. Sjogren's syndrome is a chronic inflammatory disease characterized by diminished lacrimal and salivary gland secretion. More than 90% of patients are women with a mean age of 50. The arthritis of Sjogren's syndrome resembles that of rheumatoid arthritis.

Recommended Reading

Doyle, J. R. 1993. Extensor tendons — acute injuries. *In:* Operative hand surgery, 3rd Ed., ed. D. P. Green, 1948.

Feldon, P., L. H. Millender, and E. A. Nalebuff. 1993. Rheumatoid arthritis in the hand and wrist. *In:* Operative hand surgery, 3rd Ed., ed. D. P. Green, 1587.

Lesley, B. M. 1989. Rheumatoid extensor tendon ruptures. Hand Clin. 5:919.

Nalebuff, E. A. 1968. Diagnosis, classification, and management of rheumatoid thumb deformities. Bull. Hosp. Joint Dis. 29:119.

Talal, N. 1979. Sjogren's syndrome and connective tissue disease with other immunologic disorders. *In:* Arthritis and allied conditions, 9th Ed., ed. D. J. McCarthy, 810. Philadelphia: Lea & Febiger.

Terrono, A., L. H. Millender, and E. A. Nalebuff. 1990. Boutonniere rheumatoid thumb deformity. J. Hand Surg. 15:999.

Questions

A. The most common cause of a boutonniere deformity found in the rheumatoid hand is:

1. Attenuation or rupture of the central slip
2. Attenuation or rupture of the extensor digitorum communis
3. Intrinsic muscle contracture
4. Collateral ligament rupture
5. Incarceration of the flexor superficialis

B. A 51-year-old woman with rheumatoid arthritis has had an increasing deformity and decreasing function in her dominant right thumb for the past year. She has a 45° flexion deformity of the metacarpophalangeal joint which can extend passively to neutral. She has a 50° fixed hyperextension deformity of the interphalangeal joint. Radiographs show good joint space and articular surfaces of the metacarpophalangeal joint, but significant destruction of the interphalangeal joint. The carpometacarpal joint is normal. Recommended treatment should consist of:

1. Soft tissue release/reconstruction of the thumb IP and MCP joint
2. Thumb IP and MCP joint arthrodesis
3. Thumb IP joint arthrodesis and transfer of the extensor pollicis longus to the base of the proximal phalanx
4. Thumb IP joint arthrodesis and repair/reconstruction of the flexor pollicis longus
5. Silicone arthroplasty of the thumb IP joint and transfer of the extensor pollicis longus to the base of the proximal phalanx

C. A 47-year-old woman who has rheumatoid arthritis in both hands has had increasing difficulty actively flexing the PIP joint of her right ring finger. She has full passive flexion. The limited active flexion is most likely due to:

1. Intrinsic tightness
2. Flexor tenosynovitis
3. Rupture of the A4 pulley
4. Palmar subluxation of the lateral bands at the PIP joint
5. Fixation of the lateral bands over the dorsum of the PIP joint

D. A 45-year-old, right-hand-dominant woman with rheumatoid arthritis complains of increasing stiffness in her right index finger. She has normal passive motion, but active flexion is only 20° at the DIP joint and 50° at the PIP joint. There are no palpable nodules or tenderness, clinical alignment is excellent, and the neurovascular examination is normal. Radiographs reveal good joint spaces and alignment. She has been on a variety of nonsteroidal antiinflammatory medications and has had two previous injections into her finger without improvement in its motion. Recommended treatment should be:

1. Decompression of the anterior interosseous nerve
2. Intrinsic release
3. MCP joint arthroplasty and PIP joint fusion
4. Excision of the flexor digitorum profundus and the flexor digitorum superficialis tendons; staged tendon grafting
5. Flexor tenosynovectomy

E. A 50-year-old woman with rheumatoid arthritis complains of an inability to actively extend her little, ring, and long fingers. Her fingers have full passive extension. There is no tenodesis effect with passive wrist flexion. The most likely diagnosis is:

1. MCP joint dislocation
2. Extensor tendon subluxation
3. Posterior interosseous nerve palsy
4. Extensor tendon rupture
5. Intrinsic muscle contracture

F. A 45-year-old, right-hand-dominant woman with rheumatoid arthritis complains of difficulty opening her right hand. She has swelling over the dorsal aspect of her right wrist. She has no active extension at the MCP joints of the ring and little fingers. She has full passive extension of her fingers. However, her ring and little fingers remain flexed with passive wrist flexion. Radiographs reveal distal radioulnar joint space narrowing and cysts and dorsal subluxation of the distal ulna. Treatment should include:

1. Dorsal tenosynovectomy and MCP joint arthroplasties of the ring and little fingers
2. MCP joint arthroplasties and PIP joint fusions of the ring and little fingers
3. Posterior interosseous nerve decompression and dorsal tenosynovectomy
4. Dorsal tenosynovectomy, ulnar head resection, and transfer of the extensor carpi radialis longus to the extensor digiti quinti and extensor digitorum communis ring finger
5. Dorsal extensor tenosynovectomy, distal ulna resection, transfer of the extensor indicis proprius to the extensor digiti quinti, and side-to-side transfer of the extensor digitorum communis of the ring finger to the adjacent extensor digitorum communis of the long finger

G. A 53-year-old, right-hand-dominant woman has rheumatoid arthritis. Despite good medical management, she has had recurrent right dorsal wrist pain and swelling. She has active wrist flexion and extension, but is unable to pronate or supinate due to pain in the ulnar aspect of her wrist. She cannot actively extend the MCP joints of her right ring and little fingers. Her sensation is intact. She has no passive tenodesis effect with wrist flexion. Radiographs show dorsal subluxation of the distal ulna. Recommended treatment should be tenosynovectomy of the extensor tendons and:

1. Synovectomy of the wrist
2. Resection of the distal ulna
3. Resection of the distal ulna and tendon transfers
4. Resection of the distal ulna, release of the ulnar nerve at the elbow, and tendon repairs
5. Decompression of the posterior interosseous nerve

11 Tendon Transfers

Tendon transfers are performed to improve compromised motor function when repair of an injured nerve, muscle, or tendon is impossible or has failed. The force and excursion of a muscle tendon unit are important when considering a tendon transfer to restore motor function. The cross-sectional area of a muscle is most closely associated with the force of that muscle. Ideally, tendon transfers should be synergistic. Patients with a high radial nerve palsy will generally have the pronator teres, flexor carpi ulnaris, and palmaris longus muscle tendon units as available donors for tendon transfers. The Jones transfer, which was described in 1921, has been a classic combination of transfers for restoration of functional loss due to a high radial nerve palsy. These transfers include a pronator teres transfer to the extensor carpi radialis longus and extensor carpi radialis brevis tendons; the flexor carpi radialis tendon to the extensor pollicis longus, the extensor pollicis brevis, abductor pollicis longus, and extensor digitorum communis to the index finger; and the flexor carpi ulnaris tendon to the extensor digitorum communis tendon. A low median nerve palsy can result in loss of thumb opposition. To restore thumb opposition, the transfer needs to duplicate, as closely as possible, the function of the opponens pollicis muscle. The flexor digitorum sublimis tendon to the ring finger has been used to restore thumb opposition using either a tendon loop of the flexor carpi ulnaris as a pulley at the wrist crease or a window cut in the volar carpal ligament as a pulley. This will result in a line of pull directed from the pisiform toward the thumb MCP joint, which is the same as the abductor pollicis brevis. Low ulnar nerve palsies will result in compromise of fine tip and key pinch. Key pinch can be strengthened by a number of transfers, including the extensor carpi radialis longus prolonged with a tendon graft to the adductor pollicis.

Intrinsic palsy and clawing of the hand can result from a low ulnar and median nerve palsy. The course that tendon transfers should follow to actively restore intrinsic function is volar to the intermetacarpal ligaments. Insertion of tendon transfers which are stronger and subsequently hold with power the lateral bands will result in swan neck deformities. This early complication of dynamic intrinsic transfers has been addressed by utilizing the extensor digitorum quinti or a single flexor digitorum sublimis tendon and splitting the tendons, and/or adding slips to them to result in intrinsic tendon transfer from the single tendon to all of the fingers. Tendon transfers to restore active intrinsic function are the only procedures that can correct the deformity, improve grip strength, and provide simultaneous active MP and IP joint flexion in the hand. Alternatively, procedures such as a volar capsulorrhaphy will prevent hyperextension of the MP joint and therefore allow extrinsic extensor function to actively extend the IP joints.

Rupture of the extensor pollicis longus tendon can be treated nicely with an extensor indicis proprius transfer.

Patients with cerebral palsy must have good sensation, a reasonably good pattern of grasp and release, and at least normal intelligence to be good candidates for tendon transfers. Patients with cerebral palsy who have considerable spasticity and are unable to extend the fingers with the wrist in a neutral or an extended posture may be good candidates for the flexor "slide" operation. Alternatively, the Green procedure, in which the flexor carpi ulnaris is transferred to the extensor carpi radialis, may be performed to improve grasp in a patient with cerebral palsy, but the inability to extend the fingers with the wrist extended is a contraindication to this procedure. Pronation contracture is sometimes seen in patients with spasticity. Transfer of the pronator teres insertion may improve their function and lessen the pronation contracture.

A patient with C-6 functional level quadriplegia will still have the wrist extensors functional. Tenodesis of the flexor digitorum profundus and flexor pollicis longus tendons would allow him to have a grasp pattern when he actively extends his wrist. As an alternative to this passive grasp pattern, due to the tenodesis effect caused by tenodesing the flexor digitorum profundus and flexor pollicis longus muscles, the extensor carpi radialis longus could be transferred to the flexor digitorum profundus for active finger flexion. The Steindler flexorplasty can result in weak elbow flexion in a patient who has lost active elbow flexion but still has the medial epicondylar muscles, which would be transferred to the distal medial humeral shaft.

Recommended Reading

Brand, P. W. 1988. The biomechanics of tendon transfers. Hand Clin. 4:137.

Brand, P. W., R. B. Beach, and D. E. Thompson. 1981. Relative tension and potential excursion of muscles in the forearm and hand. J. Hand Surg. 6A:209.

McCarroll, H. R. 1994. Tendon transfers. Hand knowledge update text. Am. Soc. for Surg. Hand 1601–1611.

Questions

A. When choosing a muscle for a tendon transfer, it is important to know its force. The force of a muscle is most directly associated with its:

1. Amplitude of contraction
2. Fiber length
3. Excursion
4. Cross-sectional area
5. Mass

B. In a patient with a high radial nerve palsy, the best muscle to use as a transfer to restore wrist extension is the:

1. Brachioradialis
2. Pronator teres
3. Flexor carpi ulnaris
4. Flexor carpi radialis
5. Flexor digitorum sublimis

C. Which of the following muscles would be the best to use as a tendon transfer to restore thumb opposition?

1. Extensor digiti quinti
2. Extensor indicis proprius
3. Extensor pollicis longus
4. Flexor digitorum sublimis
5. Abductor digiti quinti

D. A patient with an ulnar nerve palsy has clawing of the ring finger and little finger. A dynamic tendon transfer using the extensor digiti quinti tendon is performed to correct the clawing. The path of the tendon transfer must pass:

1. Palmar to the axis of the proximal interphalangeal joint motion
2. Palmar to the transverse intermetacarpal ligament
3. Dorsal to the axis of the metacarpophalangeal joint motion
4. Ulnar to the metacarpophalangeal joint of the little finger
5. Between the bases of the fourth and fifth metacarpals

E. The purpose of the flexor origin "slide" procedure in the treatment of spastic hemiplegia is to:

1. Allow finger extension and the wrist to move to neutral
2. Allow finger flexion and wrist extension
3. Allow finger flexion and the wrist to move to neutral
4. Decompress the ulnar nerve
5. Decompress the median nerve

F. A 26-year-old man with a C$_6$ quadriplegia is interested in improving his hand function. What muscle could be transferred to give him active finger flexion?

1. Extensor carpi ulnaris
2. Extensor carpi radialis longus
3. Brachialis
4. Abductor pollicis longus
5. Flexor carpi ulnaris

12 Brachial Plexus

Brachial plexus injuries may be due to stab wounds, gunshots, or traction from motor vehicle accidents or sports injuries. Associated injuries include many types of fractures and dislocations of the shoulder girdle and neck.

The C5 and C6 nerve roots are the ones most commonly avulsed. Upper plexus injury (Erb's palsy) involves the C5 and C6 nerve roots, with or without function of the C7 nerve root. Typically, the limb is extended at the elbow, flaccid at the side of the trunk, adducted, and internally rotated.

Obstetrical brachial plexus injuries are caused by traction, usually due to fetal malposition, cephalopelvic disproportion, and the use of forceps. These birth palsies can be an upper C6 lesion (Erb's palsy), an entire plexus lesion, or a lower plexus C7-8, T1 lesion (Klumpke's palsy) (Fig. 12-1).

In whatever age patient, lower plexus injuries can be diagnosed by finding segmental sensory and motor deficits involving C8 and T1, with or without involvement of C7. Associated Horner's syndrome (ptosis [drooping of the upper eyelid], miosis [pupil contraction], anhidrosis [absence of sweating], and enophthalmos [recession of the eyeball in the orbit]) should alert the examiner to the possibility of an avulsion injury of the lower plexus.

In any brachial plexus injury, the levels of injury should be delineated (Fig. 12-2).

Also of significant importance is to establish whether the injury is supraganglionic or infraganglionic.

An injury in which the roots are avulsed from the spinal cord is important to recognize because surgical repair is impossible. It can be diagnosed in an upper plexus injury by finding segmental motor and sensory deficits involving the C5 and C6 cervical roots with paralysis of the serratus anterior, levator scapulae, and rhomboids, indicating that the lesion of the nerve roots is medial to the emergence of the long, thoracic, and dorsal scapular nerves that supply these muscles. The

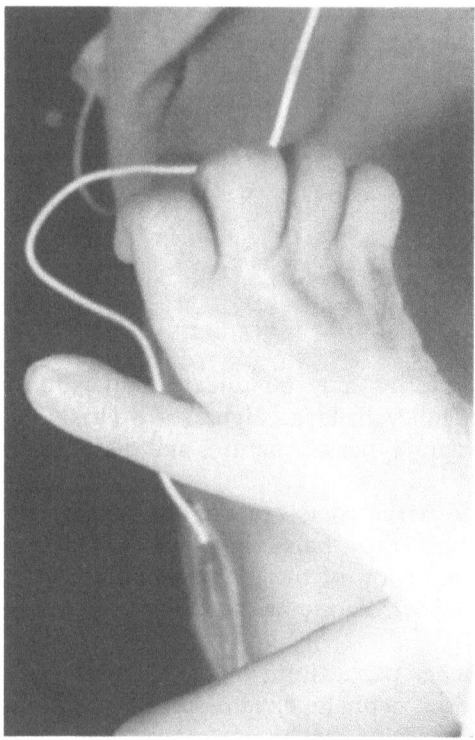

Fig. 12-1. A clinical photograph of the typical posturing of a newborn's hand with a lower brachial plexus palsy (Klumpke's palsy).

diagnosis is often confirmed by demonstrating denervation potentials in the segmental paraspinous musculature innervated by the posterior primary rami.

Myelography has been extremely helpful by demonstrating a pseudomeningocele or complete absence of root shadows. At the site of avulsion, myelography may be inaccurate soon after injury, due to occlusion of the opening of the pseudomeningocele from clotted blood. A delay of 6 to 12 weeks is suggested. MRI is now considered the preferred imaging technique. A combination of coronal and axial T2 weighted MR images can nicely demonstrate pathology and even pseudomeningocele without delay.

In differentiating preganglionic, intraspinal lesions from postganglionic, extraspinal lesions, cutaneous axon reflexes have been found to be useful. These reflexes are elicited by placing a drop of histamine on the skin. Normally, a sequential response consisting of cutaneous vasodilitation, wheal formation, and flare response occurs. If the nerve is interrupted proximal to the axon, the skin will be anesthetic, but a

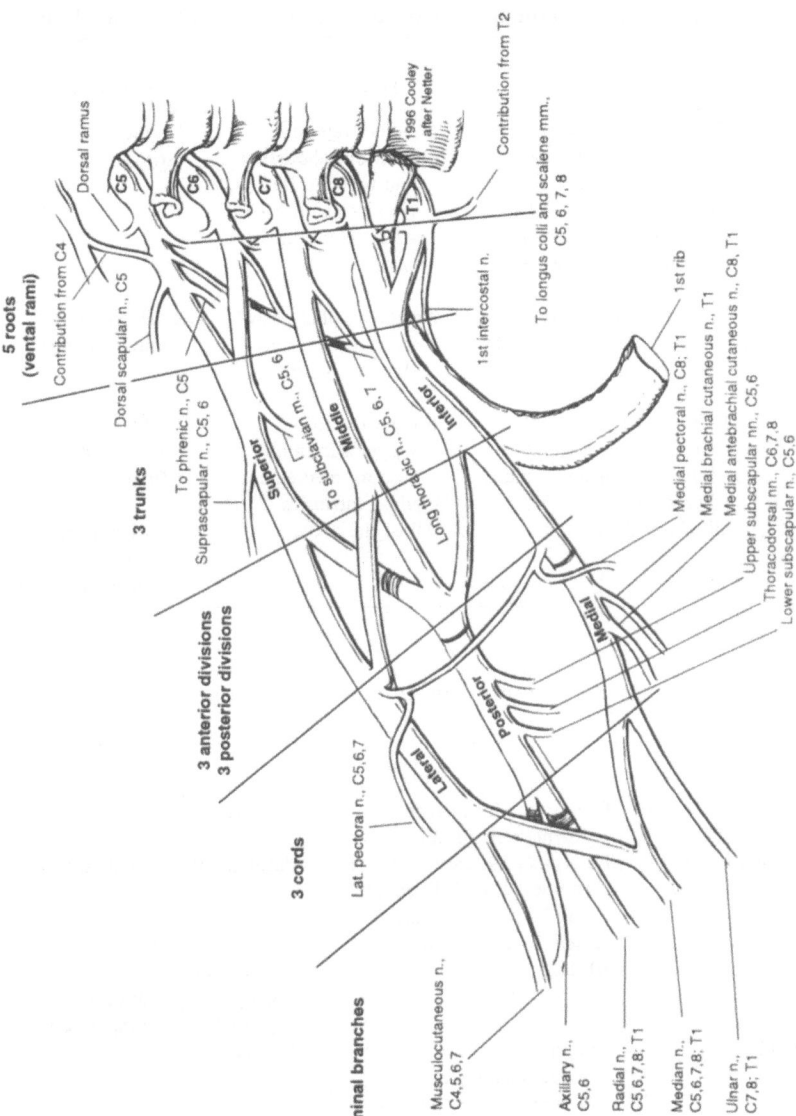

5 roots
(vental rami)

Contribution from C4

Dorsal ramus

C5

Dorsal scapular n., C5

C6

To phrenic n., C5

C7

Suprascapular n., C5, 6

3 trunks

Superior

To subclavian m., C5, 6

Middle

Long thoracic n., C5, 6, 7

Inferior

C8

T1

1996 Cooley
after Netter

Contribution from T2

To longus colli and scalene mm.,
C5, 6, 7, 8

1st intercostal n.

1st rib

3 anterior divisions
3 posterior divisions

Medial pectoral n., C8: T1

Medial brachial cutaneous n., T1

Medial antebrachial cutaneous n., C8, T1

Upper subscapular nn., C5,6

Thoracodorsal nn., C6,7,8

Lower subscapular n., C5,6

3 cords

Lat. pectoral n., C5,6,7

Lateral

Posterior

Medial

Terminal branches

Musculocutaneous n.,
C4,5,6,7

Axillary n.,
C5,6

Radial n.,
C5,6,7,8: T1

Median n.,
C5,6,7,8: T1

Ulnar n.,
C7,8: T1

Fig. 12-2. Anatomy of the brachial plexus.

Table 12.1. Neurologic and Functional Consequences of Brachial Plexus Injury

Roots involved	Muscles affected	Functional loss	Sensory loss
C6	Deltoid, suprasapinatus, and infraspinatus, biceps, brachialis, coracobrachialis, brachioradcialis, (+) radial wrist extensors, clavicular pectoralis major	Shoulder lateral rotation, abduction and forward flexion, elbow flexion, (+) wrist extension	Thumb and index finger
C6-7	As above, plus tricpes, ECRL and ECRB, FCR, EDC, EPL, EPB, and APL	As above, plus elbow, wrist, finger, and thumb extensors	As above, plus middle finger
C(7)-8, 1	(EDC, EPL) FDS, FDP, FPL, lumbricals and interossei, thenars, and hypothenars	(Finger extension) Finger and thumb flexion, median and ulnar intrinsics	(Middle finger) Little and ring fingers
C-T1	All of the above	All of the above	Anesthesia, except for medial brachium

Table 12.2. Differentiation of Supra- and Infraganglionic Lesions of the Brachial Plexus

Evaluation technique	Supraganglionic lesion	Infraganglionic lesion
Inspection	Flail arm, winged scapula, Horner's syndrome	Flail arm
Manual muscle testing	Paralysis of serratus anterior, rhomboid, (+) diaphragm, and limb musculature	Paralysis of limb musculature
Sensation	Absent in involved dermatome	Absent in involved dermatome
Tinel's sign	Absent	Present (unless supraganglionic lesions are present at the same level)
Myelography	Traumatic pseudomeningoceles, obliteration of root detail	Normal
EMG	Paravertebral muscle and limb muscle denervation	Limb muscle denervation
Nerve conduction	Motor conduction absent, (+) sensory conduction	Motor and sensory conduction absent
Axon response	Normal. Absent if infraganglionic lesion is present at the same level	Absent

normal axon response will occur. If the injury is distal to the ganglion, there is also anesthesia of the skin, and vasodilitation and wheal formation are seen, but there is no flare response.

Electromyography 3 to 4 weeks after injury is also helpful in assessing the level of injury.

Leffert emphasizes the poor prognosis after lower plexus injuries. Upper plexus infraclavicular injuries, however, have a remarkably good prognosis.

The flail anesthetic arm that may result from a brachial plexus injury is a grave problem. There are three ways to treat this: active treatment; surgical reconstruction often with a combination of fusions, tenodesis, and transfers; and amputation.

Injuries of the cords produce fairly regular patterns of altered function. Injuries of the *lateral cord* cause motor and sensory deficits in the distribution of the musculocutaneous nerve (paralysis of the biceps) and lateral root of the median nerve (paralysis of the flexor carpi radialis and pronator teres). Glenohumeral subluxation may result. This may be prevented by an aggressive program of rehabilitation of the remaining intact musculature. A sensory deficit can be detected over the anterolateral aspect of the forearm in the relatively small autonomous zone of the musculocutaneous nerve. Injuries of the *posterior cord* cause motor and sensory deficits in the distribution of the following nerves: the subscapular (paralysis of the subscapularis and teres major), the thoracodorsal (paralysis of the latissimus dorsi), the axillary (paralysis of the deltoid and teres minor), and the radial nerve (paralysis of extension of the elbow, wrist, and fingers). The disability consists mainly of the inability to internally rotate the shoulder, elevate the limb, and extend the forearm and hand. Sensory loss is most often apparent only in the autonomous zone of the axillary nerve overlying the deltoid muscle. Injuries of the *medial cord* produce the motor deficit of a combined ulnar and median nerve lesion (except for the flexor carpi radialis and pronator teres) and extensive sensory loss along the medial aspect of the arm and hand.

Recommended Reading

Hershman, E. B. 1990. Brachial plexus injuries. Clin. Sports Med. 9:311.

Leffert, R. D. 1993. Brachial plexus. *In:* Operative hand surgery, ed. D. P. Green, 1483. New York: Churchill Livingstone.

Robertson, W. C. Jr., P. L. Eichman, and W. G. Clancy. 1979. Upper trunk brachial plexopathy in football players. JAMA 241:1480.

Questions

A. A high school defensive end developed immediate pain, tingling, and weakness down his right arm upon tackling an opponent during a football game. The tingling resolved quickly while the weakness did not resolve until the next day. Radiographs of the cervicle spine are normal. The patient complains of persistent pain of the neck and right shoulder 1 week after the injury. Physical examination reveals no neurologic abnormalities, and the shoulder examination is normal. The most likely diagnosis is:

1. Traction injury of the axillary nerve
2. Long thoracic nerve
3. Upper trunk of the brachial plexus
4. Middle trunk of the brachial plexus
5. Lower trunk of the brachial plexus

B. The most common origin of the suprascapular nerve is:

1. The C5 nerve root
2. The C6 nerve root
3. The upper trunk of the brachial plexus
4. The lateral cord of the brachial plexus
5. The long thoracic nerve

C. An 18-year-old male is in a car accident and has a contusion of his forehead. He complains of neck and right shoulder pain. Physical examination demonstrates limited motion of the cervicle spine, diffuse neck and shoulder tenderness, and decreased sensation to light touch in his right thumb and index finger. He has weakness of elbow flexion and forearm supination against resistance. Radiographs are unremarkable. The most likely diagnosis is an injury to the:

1. Sixth cervical nerve root
2. Upper trunk of the brachial plexus
3. Posterior division of the middle trunk of the brachial plexus
4. Lateral cord of the brachial plexus
5. Musculocutaneous nerve

D. Most commonly, a patient with a thoracic outlet syndrome is a woman of childbearing age with poor muscular development who presents with a neurologic deficit similar to that of a compression of the:

1. Posterior interosseous nerve at the supinator muscle
2. Radial nerve in the radial groove of the humerus
3. Median nerve in the carpal tunnel
4. Ulnar nerve at the elbow
5. Ulnar nerve in Guyon's canal

E. Which of the following nerve roots contribute to the medial cord of the brachial plexus:

1. Fifth, sixth, and seventh cervical nerve roots
2. Sixth, seventh, and eighth cervical nerve roots
3. Seventh and eighth cervical nerve roots
4. Seventh and eighth cervical and first thoracic nerve roots
5. Eighth cervical and first thoracic nerve roots

F. A newborn sustains a brachial plexus injury resulting from a difficult delivery. Which of the following suggests a poor prognosis for recovery?

1. Horner's syndrome
2. Absence of reflexes
3. Associated clavicular fracture
4. Motor involvement below the elbow
5. Complete motor paralysis with intact sensation

G. A weightlifter presents with winging of the scapula. The most likely cause is an injury to the:

1. Axillary nerve
2. Suprascapular nerve
3. Spinal accessory nerve
4. Thoracodorsal nerve
5. Long thoracic nerve

13 Anatomy

Muscular Anatomy

Upper Arm

The musculature of the dorsal brachium is comprised of the three heads of the triceps and anconeus. They act to extend the elbow. The triceps muscle heads are innervated by the radial nerve. The anconeus is innervated by the nerve to the medial head of the triceps.

The anterior brachium musculature consists of the coracobrachialis, biceps brachii, and brachialis. The coracobrachialis and biceps are innervated by the musculocutaneous nerve. The brachialis is dually innervated by the musculocutaneous and radial nerves.

Forearm

The volar superficial layer of muscles originates from the common flexor origin at the medial epicondyle. This layer includes, from radial to ulnar, the pronator teres, flexor carpi radialis (which inserts on the trapezial crest or tuberosity, index metacarpal and long metacarpal), palmaris longus, and flexor carpi ulnaris. All are innervated by the median nerve, except the flexor carpi ulnaris which is innervated by the ulnar nerve.

The intermediate muscular layer is composed of the flexor digitorum superficialis, which is innervated by the median nerve.

The deep muscular layer consists of the flexor digitorum profundus, flexor pollicis longus, and pronator quadratus. The flexor profundus to the fourth and fifth fingers is innervated by the ulnar nerve. The profundus to the index and long fingers, as well as the flexor pollicis longus and pronator quadratus, is innervated by the anterior interosseous branch of the median nerve. The pronator teres and pronator quadratus are the primary pronators of the forearm.

The superficial layer of the dorsal forearm musculature includes the brachioradialis and extensor carpi radialis longus, both of which originate above the elbow along the lateral supracondylar ridge of the humerus and are innervated by the radial nerve proximal to its division into the posterior interosseous nerve. The extensor carpi radialis brevis, extensor digitorum communis, extensor digiti quinti, and extensor carpi ulnaris originate from the common extensor origin at the lateral epicondyle of the humerus and are innervated by the posterior interosseous nerve, which is a branch of the radial nerve. The radial nerve migrates toward the radius in supination and away from the radius in pronation.

The deep layers of the dorsal forearm musculature include the supinator, abductor pollicis longus, extensor pollicis brevis, extensor pollicis longus, and extensor indicis proprius, all of which are also innervated by the posterior interosseous nerve. The biceps brachii, brachioradialis, and supinator provide supination of the forearm (Fig. 13-1A).

Intrinsic Musculature of the Hand

The intrinsic muscles of the hand are composed of the palmaris brevis, which is the only motor unit supplied by the superficial branch of the ulnar nerve; the hypothenar muscles, which are innervated by the deep branch of the ulnar nerve; the thenar muscles, which are supplied by the recurrent branch of the first common palmar digital ramus of the median nerve, with the exception of the deep head of the flexor pollicis brevis, which is supplied by the deep branch of the ulnar nerve; the adductor pollicis, which is supplied by the deep branch of the ulnar nerve; the lumbricals; and the interossei. Four lumbricals are present and originate from the flexor digitorum profundus tendon near the distal end of the flexor retinaculum. These four lumbricals course distally along the radial aspect of the second through fifth digits, passing volar to the deep transverse metacarpal ligament to cross the metacarpophalangeal (MCP) joint; they then course dorsally along the radial side of the proximal phalanx to join the interossei to form the lateral band. The tendon passes volar to the axis of rotation of the MCP joint and dorsal to the axis of rotation of the proximal interphalangeal and dorsal interphalangeal joints, and thus serves as a flexor at the MCP joint and an extensor at the interphalangeal joints. The lumbricals to the index and long fingers are innervated by the second and third common proper digital rami (digital sensory branches) of the median nerve. The lumbricals to the fourth and fifth digits are innervated by the deep branch of the ulnar nerve. There are four dorsal and four volar interossei which likewise act as flexors of the MP joint with a direct insertion into the sagittal bands and volar plate as well as the base of the proximal phalanx. They course dorsally to form the lateral bands which extend the IP joints. Additionally, the dorsal interossei abduct the fingers away from the midline (axis of the third digit), and the palmar interossei adduct the digits. All of the interossei are innervated by the deep branch of the ulnar nerve (Fig. 13-1B).

Neural Anatomy

The musculocutaneous nerve is a branch of the lateral cord of the brachial plexus derived chiefly from C5 and C6, with some contribution from C4 and C7. It travels approximately 6 to 8 cm inferior to the tip of the coracoid process to lie lateral to the axillary artery in the fossa. It then pierces the coracobrachialis and passes distally between the biceps and brachialis along their lateral border. It terminates as the lateral antebrachial cutaneous nerve as it courses radially to exit beneath the biceps, and runs in an oblique manner beneath the brachioradialis and supplies sensation to the lateral aspect of the forearm.

The medial antebrachial cutaneous nerve originates from the medial cord of the brachial plexus and contains fibers from C8 and T1. It travels along the medial brachium to pierce the fascia in the distal brachium and supplies the medial aspect of the brachium as well as the medial aspect of the forearm.

The ulnar nerve is a branch of the medial cord of the brachial plexus and contains fibers from C8 and T1. In the axilla, it lies between the axillary artery and vein. In the proximal brachium, it lies on the medial side of the brachial artery. At the level of the coracobrachialis insertion, it pierces the medial intermuscular septum, accompanied by the superior ulnar collateral artery, and runs in a groove in the medial head of the triceps to the cubital tunnel. As it courses distally between the two heads of the flexor carpi ulnaris, it comes to lie on the flexor digitorum profundus and is covered by the flexor carpi ulnaris. At the junction of the proximal and middle third of the forearm, it is joined by the ulnar artery, which courses with it to the wrist on the radial side of the nerve. In the middle to distal third of the forearm, the ulnar nerve lies on the flexor digitorum profundus and between the flexor digitorum superficialis and flexor carpi ulnaris. It provides no innervation proximal to the elbow. It gives off an articular branch to the elbow joint in the area of the cubital tunnel and provides motor branches to the flexor carpi ulnaris and flexor digitorum profundus to the ulnar two digits. At the midforearm level, a palmar cutaneous branch is present which courses anterior to the ulnar artery into the palm to supply sensation to the hypothenar area. A dorsal sensory branch divides approximately 5 cm proximal to the wrist and courses beneath the flexor carpi ulnaris to route dorsally, crossing onto the dorsum of the hand near the ulnar styloid and providing sensory innervation to the ulnar aspect of the dorsum of the hand and the ulnar one and one-half digits. The nerve continues to the wrist, lying between the flexor carpi ulnaris and flexor digitorum superficialis on the medial side of the artery, and divides into deep and superficial branches as it passes to the radial side of the pisiform. The deep branch accompanies the deep branch of the artery through the interval between the abductor digiti minimi and flexor digiti

A

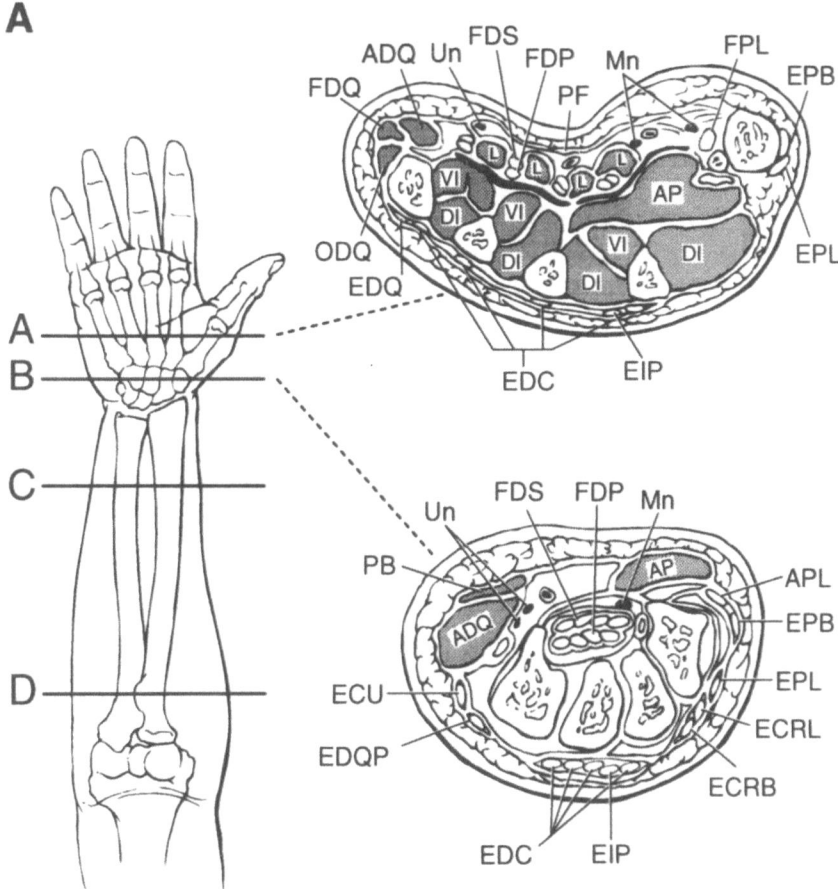

Fig. 13-1. A series of drawings of the cross-sectional anatomy at various levels of the forearm and hand. (ADQ, abductor digiti quinti; APB, abductor pollicis brevis; AP, adductor pollicis; APL, abductor pollicis longus; EDC, extensor digitorum communis; EDQ, extensor digiti quinti; EDQP, extensor digiti quinti proprius; EIP, extensor indicis proprius; EPB, extensor pollicis brevis; EPL, extensor pollicis longus; FDQ, flexor digiti quinti; FDQB, flexor digiti quinti brevis; FDP, flexor digitorum profundus; FDS, flexor digitorum sublimis; FPB, flexor pollicis brevis; FPL, flexor pollicis longus; DI, dorsal interossei; VI, volar interossei; L, lumbrical; ODQ, opponens digiti quinti; OP, opponens pollicis; PB, palmaris brevis; PF, palmar fascia; PL, palmaris longus; Br, brachioradialis; ECRL, extensor carpi radialis longus; ECRB, extensor carpi radialis brevis; ECU, extensor carpi ulnaris; FCR, flexor carpi radialis; FCU, flexor carpi ulnaris; PQ, pronator quadratus; PT, pronator teres; S, supinator; A, anconeous; Mn, median nerve; Un, ulnar nerve; Rn, radial nerve; PIn, posterior interosseous nerve.)

B

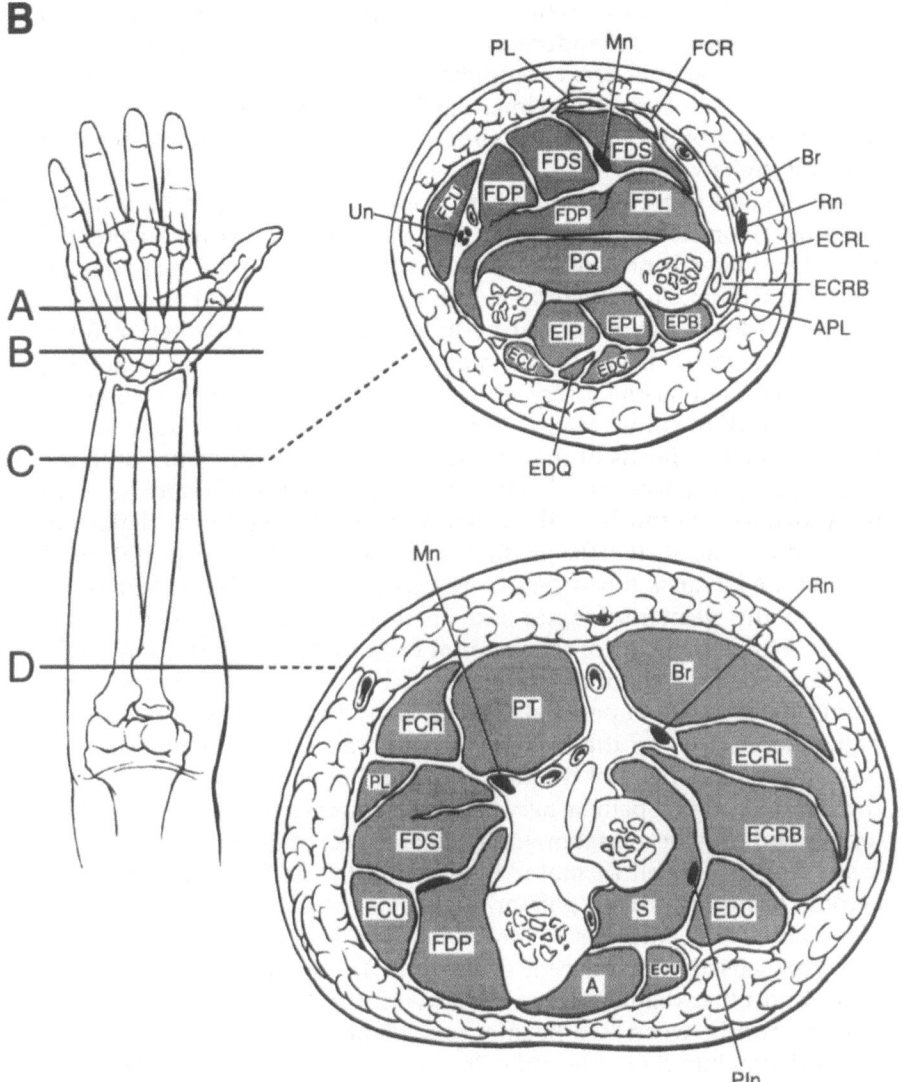

Fig. 13–1. (cont'd)

minimi brevis, and through fibers of the opponens digiti minimi to reach the deep surface of the tendons of the flexor digitorum profundus in the palm. The superficial branch supplies motor to the palmaris brevis. It then divides into common palmar digital branches and, in turn, proper palmar digital branches, which supply sensation to the ulnar one and one-half digits volarly.

The median nerve contains fibers from C6, C7, C8, and T1, with an occasional contribution from C5, and is formed by trunks from the medial and lateral cords of the brachial plexus. In the proximal one-half of the brachium, it lies lateral to the brachial artery and beneath the medial border of the biceps. At midbrachium, it crosses anterior to the brachial artery to lie along its medial side to the elbow. Following division of the brachial artery in the antecubital fossa, it lies along the medial side of the ulnar artery. As it exits the antecubital fossa, it passes between the two heads of the pronator teres and crosses anterior to the ulnar artery, which courses beneath both heads of the pronator teres. In the proximal two-thirds of the forearm, it lies on the flexor digitorum profundus beneath the flexor digitorum superficialis and in the distal third of the forearm. It becomes more superficial beneath the deep fascia between the palmaris longus and flexor digitorum superficialis as it courses beneath the flexor retinaculum volar to the profundus tendon. It divides into three common palmar digital nerves, which pass into the palm dorsal to the superficial palmar arch. The first common palmar digital nerve gives off the recurrent motor branch to the thenar muscles (except the deep head of the flexor pollicis brevis). It then divides into three proper digital palmar nerves, which course over the flexor pollicis longus and provide sensation to the volar aspect of the thumb and radial index finger, as well as motor innervation to the first lumbrical. The second common proper palmar digital nerve supplies motor to the second lumbrical and sensation to the second and third digits. The third provides sensation to adjacent sides of the third and fourth digits. The radial and ulnar digital nerves, along with the radial and ulnar digital arteries, run between two ligamentous planes. Dorsal to the neurovascular digital bundle is Cleland's ligament, and Grayson's ligament lies palmar to the neurovascular digital bundle (Fig 13-2). The branches of the median nerve include an articular branch to the elbow at the joint level and innervation to the volar forearm muscles just distal to this, as previously noted. At the level of the bicipital tuberosity of the radius, the anterior interosseous branch is given off, which runs with the anterior interosseous artery distally along the interosseous membrane to pass the pronator quadratus. The palmar cutaneous branch arises just proximal to the flexor retinaculum and runs between the flexor carpi radialis and palmaris longus to supply sensation to the thenar area and lateral palm.

The radial nerve is the largest branch of the posterior cord of the

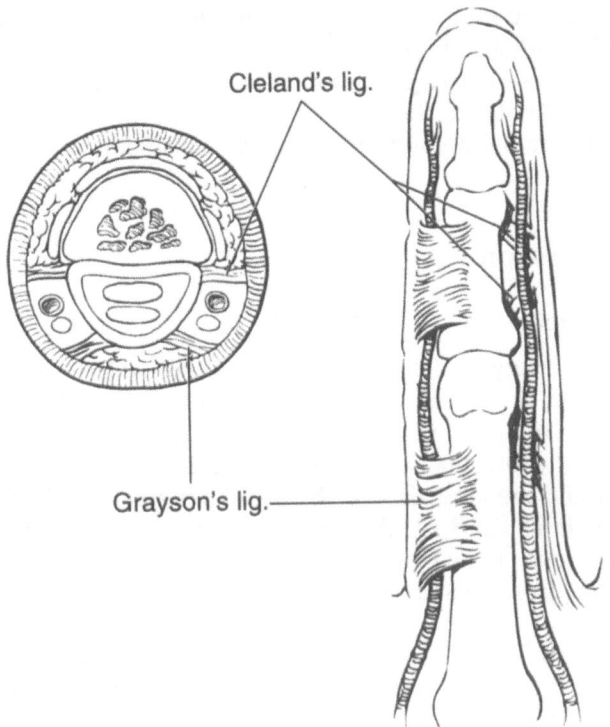

Cleland's lig.

Grayson's lig.

Fig. 13–2. Cross section through a finger, illustrating the relationship of the digital neurovascular bundles to Cleland's and Grayson's ligaments.

brachial plexus and derives fibers primarily from C6–8 and, occasionally, C4 and C5, as well as T1. It lies dorsal to the axillary artery in the axilla and then courses distally into the arm. It initially lies medial to the proximal third of the humerus and then courses directly posterior to the middle third of the humerus between the lateral and medial head of the triceps, where it is accompanied by the profunda brachii artery. At the junction of the middle and distal thirds, it courses along the musculospiral groove of the humerus to pierce the lateral intermuscular septum, and runs distally between the brachialis and brachioradialis muscles. It terminates proximal to the capitellum by dividing into the posterior interosseous nerve and superficial or sensory branch of the radial nerve. The posterior interosseous nerve runs anterior to the elbow joint in the interval between the extensor carpi radialis brevis and extensor digitorum communis to pierce the supinator. Following its exit from the supinator distally, it lies between the superficial and deep layers of the dorsal forearm musculature. It terminates as innervation to the carpal joints and passes in the radial aspect of the fourth extensor compartment. It has no cutaneous sensory component. The superficial sensory branch passes anterior to the elbow joint and descends distally behind the brachial radialis. In the distal third of the forearm, it emerges dorsally to course between the brachioradialis and flexor carpi radialis longus. It terminates in the sensory branches to the lateral thenar area, as well as the radial dorsum of the hand and digits.

Vascular Anatomy

Brachial Artery

The brachial artery is the continuation of the axillary artery from the inferior border of the teres major to its bifurcation opposite the radial neck distally. It lies on the intermuscular septum proximally to course distally on the brachialis, covered medially by the coracobrachialis proximally and then the biceps. The median nerve is lateral to the artery in the proximal third of the brachium and crosses anterior in the midbrachial level, to lie medial to the artery in the antecubital fossa. The biceps aponeurosis lies anterior and lateral to the artery at the antecubital fossa.

The profunda brachii artery branches from the brachial artery as a single trunk from the posterolateral aspect of the vessel inferior to the tendon of the teres major. It passes posterior to the brachial artery to the musculospiral groove of the humerus between the lateral and medial head of the triceps. It accompanies the radial nerve as it passes around the groove and terminates as a middle collateral and radial collateral artery. The middle collateral pierces the medial head of the triceps to anastomose with the interosseous recurrent artery at the elbow. The radial collateral courses between the brachialis and brachioradialis to anastomose with the radial recurrent artery deep to the brachioradialis. The superior and inferior ulnar collateral vessels arise from the midaspect of the brachial artery and course distally to form an anastomosis at the elbow with the ulnar recurrent vessels, which branch from the ulnar artery distal to the elbow.

Ulnar Artery

The larger of the two terminal branches of the brachial artery begins at the level of the radial neck and courses beneath both heads of the pronator teres and flexor digitorum superficialis to the ulnar side of the proximal forearm, where it proceeds distally under the flexor carpi ulnaris with the flexor digitorum profundus dorsal to it and the flexor digitorum superficialis on its lateral side. It courses superficial to the flexor retinaculum on the radial side of the ulnar nerve to pass to the radial side of the pisiform beneath the pisohamate ligament, where it divides into two branches. The superficial branch lies deep to the palmaris brevis and hypothenar fascia. It courses toward the radial side deep to the palmar fascia and superficial to the flexor tendons and digital branch of the ulnar and median nerves to form a superficial palmar arch, which it completes radially by anastomosing with the superficial palmar branch of the radial artery or by union with the deep palmar arch by way of the princeps pollices artery. The superficial arch gives off three common digital arteries, which pass through the palm beside the flexor tendon volar to the digital nerve and lumbricals. They unite with the palmar metacarpal arteries from the deep palmar arch and bifurcate to form proper digital arteries to the adjacent side of the digits.

Radial Artery

The radial artery begins at the level of the radial head lying anterior to the biceps tendon and courses laterally to the supinator, proceeding distally along the pronator teres in the proximal forearm, to which it is most bound by fascia. In the proximal forearm, it is covered by the brachioradialis and proceeds distally to lie lateral to the flexor carpi radialis and medial to the brachioradialis and superficial branch of the radial nerve. The radial recurrent artery arises from the lateral side of the radial artery just distal to its origin and courses laterally across the supinator. Branches extend between the brachialis and brachioradialis proximally to accompany the radial nerve and anastomose with the radial collateral branch of the profunda brachii artery, which supplies the elbow joint and surrounding musculature. This vessel is vulnerable to injury with anterior and anterolateral surgical approaches. At the wrist, the radial artery courses dorsally distal to the radial styloid to lie deep to the tendons of the first and third extensor compartments. It runs dorsal to the scaphoid and trapezium, and enters the palm between the base of the first and second metacarpals through the interval between the two heads of the first dorsal interosseous. Initially, it lies between the first dorsal interosseous and adductor pollicis on the volar aspect of the second metacarpal base. It proceeds ulnarward on the volar surface of the interossei, accompanied by the deep branch of the ulnar nerve. On the ulnar side of the palm, it joins the deep ulnar artery to form the deep palmar arch, which lies approximately 1.5 cm proximal to the superficial arch and lies dorsal to the flexor tendons. Branches of the deep palmar arch include the princeps pollicis and radialis indicis arteries. The princeps pollices arises in the palm between the first dorsal interosseous and adductor pollicis and parallels the first metacarpal along its ulnar border deep to the flexor pollicis longus tendon. It divides at the level of the MP joint to form the two palmar digital arteries to the thumb. The radialis indicis runs distally between the first dorsal interosseous and adductor pollicis, and branches at the MP level to supply the radial side of the index and adjacent side of the second and third digits. The palmar metacarpal arteries are three in number and lie on the interosseous muscles, and join the palmar common digital artery from the superficial arch.

Fingertip Anatomy

The anatomy of the perionychium includes the nail bed, the dorsal roof and ventral floor of the nail fold, and the lunula (Fig. 13-3).

Clinical Correlation

Accurate assessment of clinical conditions depends on a knowledge of anatomy. There is an increasing inventory of reported anatomic variations in the upper extremity. This chapter will discuss the commonly accepted description of upper extremity anatomy. The planning of surgical exposures takes into account the structures within the field. In the upper extremity, anterior and anterolateral approach to the elbow requires vigilance to avoid injury to the radial recurrent artery, as well as the lateral antebrachial cutaneous nerve which supplies sensation to the lateral aspect of the forearm and courses obliquely toward the brachio-

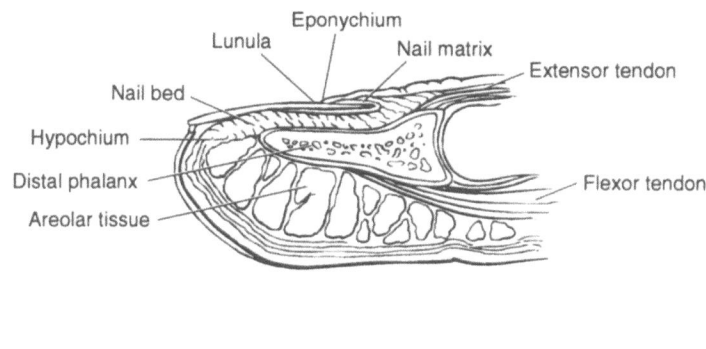

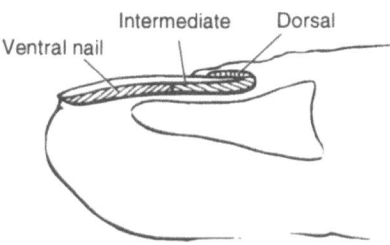

Fig. 13-3. Section through the distal fingertip illustrating the various components of a fingernail.

radialis as it exits from between the biceps and brachialis muscles. A posterior approach to the elbow that splits the triceps and forcefully retracts the medial head of the triceps jeopardizes the ulnar nerve and its distal function, as well as its most proximal branches, which innervate the flexor carpi ulnaris. A posterolateral approach, as utilized for radial head excision, jeopardizes the posterior interosseous nerve if carried too far distally. The eponym for the dorsal approach to the proximal third of the forearm is the Thompson approach, which proceeds in the interval between the extensor carpi radialis brevis and extensor digitorum communis. The posterior interosseous nerve is in jeopardy with this approach and is protected by pronation of the forearm, which moves it away from the dorsal surface of the radius. The anterior, or Henry, approach to the middle and distal third of the forearm develops the interval between the brachioradialis and flexor carpi radialis, with isolation and protection of the radial artery and retraction of it medially to expose the anterior surface of the radius. In the proximal third of the forearm, the radial artery is most closely bound by fascia to the pronator teres. For exposure of the volar digits, the Bruner volar zig-zag approach gives excellent access (Fig. 13-4).

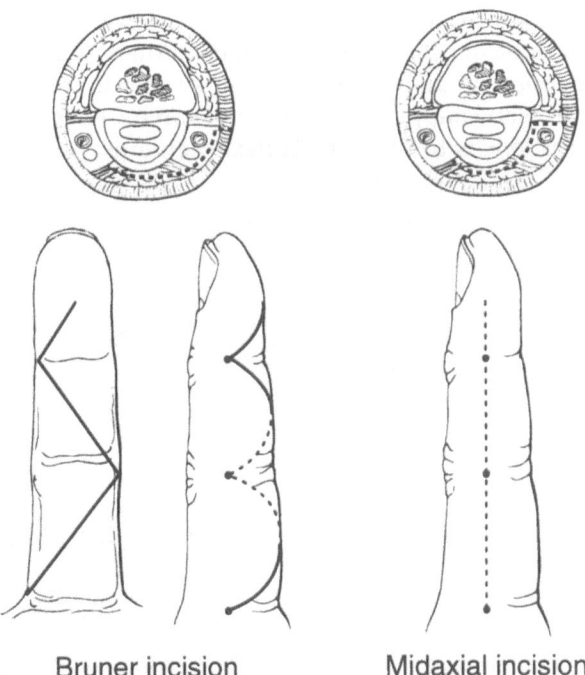

Bruner incision   Midaxial incision

Fig. 13-4. The skin incision and the dissection plane for (A) a Bruner volar zig-zag incision and (B) a midaxial incision.

Knowledge of the pathomechanics and the anatomy involved in trauma can help one predict and understand the injury and its clinical effect. The insertion of the flexor digitorum profundus tendon is to the metaphyseal region, and the extensor tendon insertion is to the epiphyseal region of the distal phalanx of the fingers in a skeletally immature child. Fracture patterns that occur with extensor tendon avulsion injuries differ between skeletally immature and mature fingers (Fig 13–5). Injury to the deep branch of the ulnar nerve causes loss of strong thumb adduction, with reduced key-pinch grip and the inability to turn a key in a lock forcefully. A volar dislocation of the proximal interphalangeal (PIP) joint of the finger is listed as resulting in disruption of the central slip of the extensor mechanism, although recent reports indicate that the rent occurs between the central slip and lateral band. Lateral displacement of the base of the first metacarpal that occurs with a Bennett's fracture is due primarily to the pull of the abductor pollicis longus. The lunula of the nail represents the distal extent of the germinal matrix, and injury to this area can result in permanent deformity.

Knowledge of vascular anatomy can help shape the preference among treatment options for specific disorders. A volar approach for bone grafting a nonunion of the scaphoid is preferred because of the lower risk of compromising the blood supply to the scaphoid in this approach than a dorsal approach. With laceration of both flexor tendons at the midproximal phalangeal level, resection of the distal cut end of the sublimis tendon will disrupt the vincular system to the profundus and jeopardize its blood supply. This is why the preferred treatment of flexor tendon lacerations is to repair both flexor tendons.

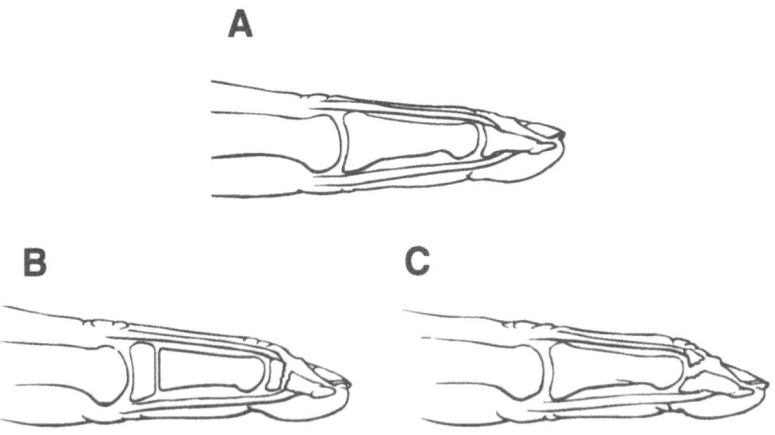

Fig. 13–5. (A) The insertion of the flexor digitorum profundus and the extensor tendon on the distal phalanx and the typical mallet finger fracture pattern in (B) a skeletally immature child and in (C) a skeletally mature adult.

Infectious processes follow anatomic planes and spaces when they spread. A purulent flexor tenosynovitis of the third, fourth, and fifth fingers that extends proximally can involve the midpalmar space. Involvement of the index finger and thumb with proximal extension would involve the thenar space. The hypothenar space contains the hypothenar muscles and rarely is involved with a deep space infection.

The most common ganglion is the dorsal wrist ganglion, whose stalk originates from the dorsal portion of the scapholunate interosseous ligament. Elbow dislocation can disrupt the medial collateral ligament, which is the most important structure for stability. Instability of the distal radioulnar joint alerts to the need for assessment of the triangular fibrocartilage complex, which is the primary static stabilizer of the joint. Insertion of proximal pins for application of an external fixator can cause injury to the superficial radial nerve in the distal third of the forearm as it courses between the brachioradialis and extensor carpi radialis longus. Proximally in the forearm, it courses beneath the brachioradialis; as it extends distally, it emerges dorsally from behind the brachioradialis tendon.

Suggested Reading

Bishop, A. T., G. Gabel, and S. W. Carmichael. 1994. The flexor carpi radialis tendonitis. Part I: Operative anatomy. J. Bone Joint Surg. A:1009.

Grant, J. C. B. 1962. Grant's atlas of anatomy. Baltimore: Williams & Wilkins.

Marble, H. C. 1961. The hand: A manual and atlas for the general surgeon. Philadelphia: W.B. Saunders Co.

Steichen, J. C., and B. W. Ellis. 1971. Vulnerability of the posterior interosseous nerve during radial head resection. J. Bone Joint Surg. 53B:320.

Warfel, J. H. 1985. The extremities: Muscles and motor points. 5th Ed. Philadelphia: Lea & Febiger.

Questions

A. During a dorsal surgical approach in a finger in which the dissection is extended lateral and volar, what ligament must be divided in order to reach the neurovascular bundles?

1. Transverse retinacular
2. Natatory
3. Skoog's
4. Cleland's
5. Grayson's

B. What portion of the nail is the lunula?

1. Junction of the sterile nail matrix with the hyponychium
2. Junction of the proximal and lateral nail folds
3. Proximal margin of the germinal nail matrix
4. Distal margin of the germinal nail matrix
5. Distal margin of the sterile nail matrix

C. In a skeletally immature child with open physes, which of the following correctly describes the flexor and extensor tendon insertions?

1. Flexor and extensor tendons inserts into metaphysis
2. Flexor and extensor tendons inserts into epiphysis
3. Flexor tendon inserts into metaphysis, extensor tendon inserts into epiphysis
4. Flexor tendon inserts into epiphysis, extensor tendon inserts into metaphysis
5. Flexor tendon inserts into epiphysis and metaphysis, extensor tendon inserts into epiphysis

D. The innervation of the lumbrical muscles to the index and long fingers is from the:

1. Terminal branches of the posterior interosseous
2. Terminal branches of the anterior interosseous
3. Deep branch of the ulnar
4. Digital sensory nerves to the index and long fingers
5. Thenar motor branch of the median

E. The primary structure for elbow joint stability is the:

1. Brachialis muscle
2. Flexor carpi ulnaris muscle
3. Medial collateral ligament
4. Lateral collateral ligament
5. Annular ligament

F. During a posterolateral surgical approach to the elbow which exposes the radial head and the annular ligament, what structure is at risk of injury with further dissection distal?

1. The common interosseous artery
2. The superficial radial nerve
3. The posterior interosseous nerve
4. The radial recurrent artery
5. The posterior interosseous artery

G. What structure passes through the lateral intermuscular septum in association with the radial nerve?

1. The anterior interosseous nerve
2. The superior ulnar collateral artery
3. The radial recurrent artery
4. The brachial artery
5. The profunda brachii artery

H. If untreated, a septic flexor tenosynovitis of the ring finger would most likely rupture into:

1. The hypothenar space
2. The thenar space
3. The mid-palmar space
4. The subaponeurotic space
5. Perona's space

14 Congenital Anomalies

Congenital amputation of the upper extremity is an uncommon deformity that is transmitted sporadically by chance mutation, with no mode of genetic transmission having been identified. It occurs approximately 10 times more commonly below the elbow than above the elbow. Clinically, the appearance of the extremity proximal to the amputation will reveal atrophy of the musculature proximal to the amputation, as opposed to amputation secondary to constrictive bands, which are normal proximally. Only rarely is operative intervention required for stump revision or removal of digital remnants for bilateral below-the-elbow amputation. Occasionally, it is necessary to perform a Krukenberg procedure on one side to convert the radius and the ulna in the forearm into a controllable pair of opposable prehensile digits.

At 4 to 6 months of age, when crawling is attempted and good sitting balance has been attained, fitting with a socket, harness, and passive mitt-type terminal device is indicated. Training for an active terminal device can be instituted at the age of 2.

Radial club hand was originally thought to be transmitted by an autosomal-dominant mode, but it now appears that environmental factors, including toxins and other chemicals, are responsible for sporadic occurrence. It is bilateral in approximately 50% of cases. It is noted that radial absence does not correlate directly with hand deficiency, but does correlate directly with instability of the hand at the wrist, as well as forearm soft tissue deficiencies (Fig. 14–1). Radial aplasia is most often associated the VATER syndrome (vertebral, anal, tracheal, esophageal, and renal defects).

Clinically, the extremity appears to have a shortened forearm bowed to the radial side, with prominence of the distal ulna (Fig. 14–2). The thumb may be hypoplastic or absent, and the MP and PIP joints of the index and long fingers may exhibit stiffness and loss of motion. Radial deviation of the hand is noted, and carpal deficiency is related to the thumb deformity, with absence of the radial carpal bones with thumb aplasia. The preaxial musculature of the forearm is atrophic, and the

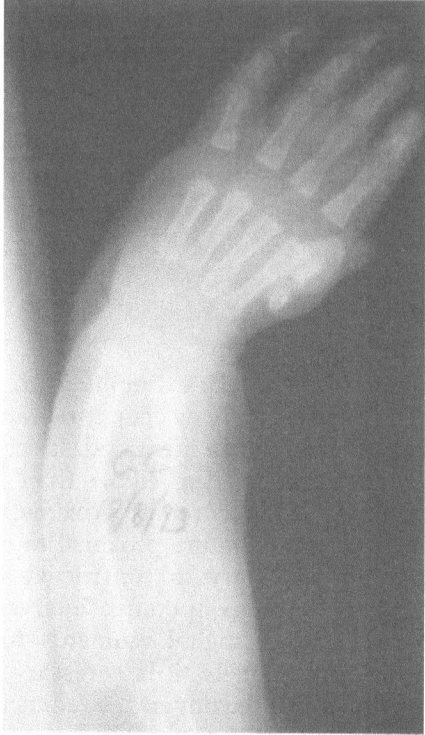

Fig. 14-1. A PA radiograph of the forearm and hand of a patient with radial club hand showing the hypoplastic radius, the longer bowed ulna, and the radially deviated posture of the hand.

thenar muscles are usually deficient. The radial artery is usually noted to be absent, with the ulnar artery being intact. The median and ulnar nerves are usually spared of involvement, but the sensory branch of the radial nerve is usually absent. The brachioradialis musculature can act as a tethering force in radial deviation of the hand.

Treatment can cover the spectrum from simple observation and essentially no treatment, to surgical intervention. Initially, serial casting is undertaken for correction of soft tissue contractures. This is instituted as a newborn. Operative treatment is generally indicated for instability of the hand, due to inadequate radial support at the wrist, thumb, and finger deformities sufficiently severe to require operative treatment, and soft tissue contracture involving the radial aspect of the wrist and forearm that are unresponsive to conservative measures. Operative treatment consists of adequate soft tissue release, in addition to centralization of the carpus over the distal ulna. Dynamic balancing with tendon transfers to resist deformity force is indicated, and capsular reefing is necessary for stabilization. An ulnar osteotomy may be

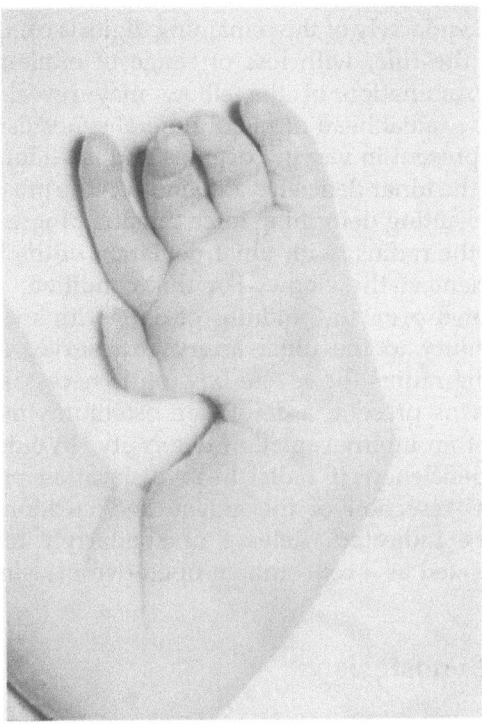

Fig. 14-2. A clinical photograph showing the typical clinical appearance of a patient with a radial club hand.

necessary to correct severe ulnar bowing. Fibular transplantation is not generally successful because the fibular transplant grows too slowly to provide continued adequate support. Operative treatment, when deemed necessary, is undertaken between 3 and 6 months of age.

Ulnar club hand is a congenital deformity of the upper extremity that occurs as a sporadic occurrence, with no known mode of genetic transmission having been identified. Ulnar club hand differs from radial deficiency in that ulnar deficiency is more likely to be partial than totally absent, as is radial deficiency. The ulnar deficiency presents with a stable wrist and an unstable elbow, as opposed to a radial deficiency, which presents primarily with instability of the carpus. Associated abnormalities with ulnar deficiency involve primarily the muscular system and include radial head dislocation, radiohumeral synostosis, club foot, and fibular deficiency. Hand defects are noted to be more common with ulnar deficiencies, as opposed to radial deficiencies, and may involve any digit.

Clinically, the forearm appears to be short and is curved to the ulnar side. The hand is deviated toward the ulnar side, and the ulnar one to three digits may be absent, with corresponding carpal bone absence being present. Syndactyly of the remaining digits is common, and elbow involvement is the rule, with loss of range of motion being present. Radiographic examination of the elbow may reveal subluxation or dislocation of the radial head or radiohumeral synostosis. The proximal ulna is usually present in varying degrees and is seldom totally absent.

Treatment of the ulnar deficiency depends on the presence of an ulnar anlage and its resulting deforming force causing progressive shortening and bowing of the radius, with ulnar deviation of the hand and radial head displacement at the elbow. For this condition, resection of the anlage is indicated prior to 6 months of age, with special attention to avoidance of injury to the ulnar artery and nerve. Occasionally, an osteotomy of the radius for severe bowing is necessary. If a radiohumeral synostosis is present, a derotation osteotomy may be necessary for correction of an internal rotation deformity. In older children with type II ulnar deficiency, if radial head dislocation precludes normal elbow function, resection of the anlage and creation of a one-bone forearm may be indicated. Release of syndactyly for the hand, as needed, is indicated as a concomitant operative measure.

Radioulnar Synostosis

Synostosis most commonly occurs in the forearm proximally. Two types are present. Type I is usually complete and occurs in the proximal aspect of the forearm. Type II is more likely to be incomplete and occurs just distal to the proximal radial epiphysis. This type is not uncommonly associated with radial head dislocations.

Most cases occur as isolated or random incidences, but some familial case reports are present. The deformity may be a component of syndromes, especially acrocephalosyndactyly. It also may be present in autosomal chromosomal aberrations as well as sex chromosomal abnormalities, especially Klinefelter's syndrome and its variants. Associated anomalies include general skeletal abnormalities including CDH, club foot, and preaxial hand deformities.

A pronation or hyperpronation deformity is the common presenting clinical picture with associated hypoplastic soft tissues.

Treatment is directed toward patients only if symptomatic or with significant loss of function. Present evidence indicates that surgical intervention does not markedly improve function, and more emphasis is being placed on nonoperative treatment. It is recognized that the patient is functionally disabled if the deformity is bilateral or is greater than 45° and pronation is present. Attempts to take down the synostosis have proven to be futile, and at present the procedure of choice is an osteotomy performed proximally through the level of the synostosis. Timing of the surgical procedure should be prior to 10 years of age, as circulatory embarrassment is less common when performed at that time. It is recommended when the osteotomy is performed that the deformity be corrected to mild pronation of less than 25° or to supination on one side if the deformity is bilateral. The more distal the osteotomy is performed, the greater the risk of neurovascular embarrassment.

Clinodactyly

This deformity refers to deviation of a digit in the coronal plane resulting from abnormal angulation of either IP joint due to arrested development usually of the middle phalanx. This most commonly involves the fifth digit and is represented by radial deviation at the DIP joint and has an associated hypoplastic middle phalanx. It is known to be associated with a multitude of syndromes and has been postulated to be a possible indicator of mental retardation.

Treatment is reserved for loss of function which is rare or more commonly for cosmesis. Osteotomy of the middle phalanx, either opening or closing wedge, is usually the procedure of choice and is not indicated prior to age 6 years.

Kirner's Deformity

This deformity is represented by radiovolar curvature of the distal phalanx of the fifth digit with widening of the epiphysis that first becomes apparent in childhood and progresses with growth. It is usually bilateral and symptomatic.

Splinting may provide symptomatic relief but does not alter the progression of the process. Operative treatment, when indicated, consists of multiple osteotomies with axial pin fixation.

Trigger Digit

This deformity has two presentations—an infantile presentation and a childhood presentation. The patient commonly presents with a flexed distal joint but, less commonly, can present with a distal joint fixed in extension. Palpable clicking with range of motion may be palpable, and difficulty with passive extension of the flexed DIP joint may be present. Spontaneous resolution of the condition occurs more frequently in the infantile form of trigger digit than in the childhood presentation. The long-term adverse effect of the condition is fixed joint contracture at the DIP joint. There appears to be familial incidence, but no known mode of genetic transmission has been identified. It is noted to occur in trisomy 13 syndrome, known as Patau's syndrome.

Spontaneous resolution can occur in approximately one-third of cases of infantile presentation and in about 10% of childhood cases. With regard to treatment, splinting appears to be of no benefit, and operative relief by age 3 is noted to prevent permanent flexion contracture. The operative procedure of choice is identical for the same condition in the adult.

Congenital Ulnar Drift

This deformity presents with ulnar deviation of the digits that progresses with growth. The most disabling component of this deformity is the marked adduction of the thumb to the palm. Associated soft tissue abnormalities including dislocation of the extensor mechanism are present. Associated findings include flexion contracture at the MP and occasionally the IP joints, as well as limitation of rotation of the forearm. Associated abnormalities include limb girdle abnormalities with thoracic and shoulder involvement, as well as scoliosis. Foot deformities and facial deformities also accompany this condition.

Treatment recommendations include early splinting, but this is not markedly beneficial. Operative intervention includes soft tissue procedures such as releases as well as extensor tendon relocation and possible tendon transfers. Operative timing is approximately age 6 years. Adults with this condition require osteotomy for correction of their deformities.

Delta Phalanx

This is characterized by the abnormal semilunar shape of the proximal epiphysis of the involved bone, which causes progressive angulation. Clinical appearance is deviation inward of the border digits. It can be associated with other hand deformities, as well as Apert syndrome, Poland's, and Holt-Oram syndrome.

Associated abnormalities affect the surgical treatment. In general, the isolated condition in the central digits is allowed to skeletally mature with age. A wedge osteotomy is used as a method to correct angular deformities. In children, deformities may recur following operative procedure as growth progresses and may need to be repeated. Arthrodesis or amputation for nonfunctional digits may be necessary in the adult.

Madelung's

Madelung's deformity is a genetic defect that can occur as an isolated wrist deformity or as a manifestation of dyschondrosteosis (LERI-WEILL disease). The distal forearm deformity is the same in both, but dyschondrosteosis has other associated skeletal abnormalities. Madelung's deformity is seen in several generalized congenital abnormalities including sex chromosomal abnormalities (Turner's syndrome) and other skeletal dysplasias.

Pathologically, the condition is characterized by a growth abnormality of the ulnar and volar half of the distal radial epiphysis that results in inclination of the radial articular surface and subsequent shift of the carpus volar with the ulna remaining dorsal. This results in the characteristic deformity, as well as loss of wrist and forearm motion, especially extension and supination. This does not become clinically apparent until middle to late childhood and presents with the characteristic deformity as described above with the prominent dorsal ulna. The forearm may be short.

Primary indication for treatment is pain. Function is usually satisfactory, as the patients can generally accommodate well for the deformity and loss of motion. If pain persists, it is usually caused by ulnocarpal impingement and is addressed by excision or shortening of the elongated distal ulna. The angular deformity of the distal radius can be treated by epiphysiodesis of the radial portion of the physis, corrective biplanar osteotomy, or physeal arrest of the ulnar half of the distal radial physis as dictated by deformity and patient age.

Congenital Clasped Thumb

This deformity can be a result of deficiency of the extensor pollicis longus, extensor pollicis brevis, or abductor pollicis longus. The clinical presentation and treatment are determined by the anatomic structure involved.

Normally, a clasped thumb posture is present for the first 3 to 4 months of life, after which time hand patterns are beginning to be established and the thumb is taken from the clutched palm position. With this deformity there is adduction of the first metacarpal with varying degrees of flexion at the MP and IP joint of the thumb, depending on the structures involved. The most common associated abnormality is club foot. Treatment is obviously determined by the structure involved. Generally, if the deformity is supple and unilateral, nonoperative treatment can be attempted with stretching, casting, and splinting of the soft tissues of the web space, and this is usually successful. If structures are deficient, surgery may be necessary in the form of soft tissue releases, tendon transfers, or arthrodesis. The tendon transfer utilized for extensor pollicis longus deficiency includes use of the brachioradialis, palmaris longus, or extensor carpi radialis longus. The most consistent pathologic finding in congenital clasped thumb is hypoplasia or absence of the extensor pollicis brevis. The extensor indicis proprius is the ideal motor unit for transfer as it is usually normal and unaffected by the process. When the deformity is seen following skeletal maturity, arthrodesis of the MP joint with extensor indicis proprius transfer to the EPL is the treatment of choice. Prior to any definitive tendon transfer or bone procedure, adequate soft tissue stretching and/or relief must be accomplished to allow correction of the deformity.

Hypoplastic Thumb

This represents a developmental defect of the thumb that adversely affects hand function. The presence of associated congenital anomalies and osseous and soft tissue deficiencies dictates appropriate treatment.

A *short thumb* represents osseous hypoplasia with no significant loss of function. The phalanges or the metacarpal can be involved. No treatment is usually required.

The *adducted thumb* represents osseous and soft tissue hypoplasia with contraction of the first web space. The thenar muscles may be absent, and the flexor pollicis longus may be defective. The primary functional loss is due to the adduction contracture of thumb, and correction of the first web space contracture is necessary. If the thenar muscles are absent, tendon transfers to restore abduction and opposition are indicated as well as transfers to restore function of a deficient flexor pollicis longus.

The *abducted thumb* is represented by marked instability of the MP joint with loss of function. The first web space and the thenar muscles are usually deficient. These factors have to be addressed for correction.

The *floating thumb* is represented by a slender pedicle attached to the radial side of hand. Osseous hypoplasia with absence of the base of the first metacarpal and concomitant intrinsic and extrinsic soft tissue deficiency characterize this deformity. The digit is nonfunctional and is treated by pollicization in bilateral cases.

The *absent thumb* may have associated radial deficiencies and be associated with a multitude of syndromes. Pollicization of the index is the procedure of choice.

Macrodactyly

True macrodactyly is a rare congenital abnormality characterized by enlargement of all structures of a digit, with the index finger being the most commonly affected. Enlargement progresses with growth until skeletal maturation, and there is generally a limitation of range of motion with normal sensation at adulthood.

The etiology of this deformity is unclear, but no mode of inheritance is identified. A neuroabnormality is postulated to stimulate abnormal growth. Syndactyly and polydactyly occasionally occur, and, rarely, patients with the deformity have findings compatible with neurofibromatosis. No systemic defects are associated with deformity.

All tissues of the digit are enlarged, and proximal enlargement of the median or ulnar nerve may occur. Treatment of the childhood deformity is designed to debulk the digit and is done in two stages to avoid vascular compromise. Osteotomy for angular deformity and epiphyseodesis at the appropriate age are considered cessation of longitudinal growth. In older children and adults, bone shortening can be done to decrease size. Amputation is reserved for painful and nonfunctional digits.

Congenital Constriction Band Syndrome

This disorder is represented by band constriction associated with acral absence or acrosyndactyly with a variable amount of swelling distal to the constriction. The key feature of this disorder is that the part is normal proximal to the band.

Other deformities are associated with this disorder, such as club feet, cleft lip and palate, and cranial and nail abnormalities. Distal sensory and vascular deficits are seen with severe constriction. No visceral abnormalities are present.

Operative treatment is considered for cosmesis and functional reasons as well as relief of neurovascular compromise. Acrosyndactyly should be separated in the first 4 to 6 months of life, and the constriction band excised with Z-plasty closure should be done in two stages to avoid vascular compromise.

Suggested Reading

Dobyns, J. H., V. E. Wood, and L. G. Bayne. 1993. Congenital hand deformities. *In:* Operative hand surgery, 3rd Ed. D. P. Green, ed., 251.

Flatt, A. E. 1994. The care of congenital hand anomalies, 2nd Ed. St. Louis: Quality Medical Publishers.

Lister, G. D. 1994. Congenital. *In:* Hand surgery update, Chap. 38, 1-10. American Society for Surgery of the Hand, Englewood, CO.

Questions

A. A congenital growth disturbance to which portion of the distal radius can result in a Madelung's deformity?

1. The dorsal, ulnar portion
2. The dorsal, radial portion
3. The volar, ulnar portion
4. The volar, radial portion
5. All of the epiphysis

B. Macrodactyly is most commonly associated with:

1. Hypoplastic fibula
2. Poland's syndrome
3. Maffucci's syndrome
4. Neurofibromatosis
5. Vertebral, anal, tracheal, esophageal, and renal defects

C. A 6-month-old girl has a right radial club hand with normal right elbow motion. Treatment of her radially deviated hand should include casting and splinting, followed by:

1. Release of the extensor muscles
2. Tendon transfer for finger movement
3. Wrist arthrodesis
4. Vascularized fibular grafting to reconstruct the absent portion of the radius
5. Centralization of the carpus on the ulna

D. Camptodactyly includes which of the following abnormalities?

1. A delta phalanx with resulting radiovolar deviation of the little finger
2. Radial deviation of the index finger at the proximal interphalangeal joint
3. Flexion deformity of the proximal interphalangeal joint of the little finger
4. Contracture of the first dorsal interosseous muscle
5. Complex syndactyly of the index finger, long finger, and ring finger

E. A 10-month-old boy has bilateral thumb hypoplasia. The thumbs are small and unstable and have no active motion. Radiographs show metacarpals to be absent in each thumb. The recommended treatment of these deformities is:

1. Bone grafting to reconstruct the thumb metacarpals
2. Amputation of the thumbs
3. Amputation of the thumbs and pollicization of the index fingers
4. Amputation of the thumbs and great toe transplantation
5. Physical therapy, splinting, and observation

F. A 14-month-old child with Apert's syndrome presents with her mother for evaluation and treatment of the child's hand deformities. The child is developmentally slow and is believed to have a slight mental retardation. The child has bilateral acrosyndactyly of all fingers and independent thumbs. Recommended treatment should be:

1. No treatment
2. Observation until the child is 5 to 7 years old, then reassess the child's hand function and developmental level
3. Early separation of the fingers
4. Early amputation of the long and small fingers, allowing the index and ring fingers to be free
5. Early amputation of the fingers and use of an orthosis

G. Examination of a 2-year-old child that presents to you for evaluation reveals that she does not have any pectoral muscle on the right. The most common congenital abnormality of the hand associated with this condition is:

1. Acrosyndactyly of all the fingers on the ipsilateral side as the absent pectoral muscle
2. Bilateral hypoplastic thumbs
3. An absent fifth metacarpal on the ipsilateral side as the absent pectoral muscle
4. Hypoplastic thumb on the ipsilateral side in which the pectoral muscle is absent
5. Hypoplasia of the hand and simple syndactyly of the fingers on the ipsilateral side as the absent pectoral muscle

H. A 4-year-old boy is seen with a congenital posterior-lateral dislocation of the head of the radius. Treatment should best be:

1. Immediate closed reduction and cast immobilization
2. Open reduction and reconstruction of the annular ligament
3. Shortening of the proximal radius and reduction of the radial head onto the capitellum at 8 to 10 years of age
4. No treatment or radial head excision following skeletal maturity
5. Elbow arthroplasty following skeletal maturity

I. Which one of the following is most commonly associated with radial aplasia?

1. Neurofibromatosis
2. Ollier's disease
3. Poland's syndrome
4. Hypoplastic fibula
5. Vertebral, anal, tracheal, esophageal, and renal defects

15 Miscellaneous

Dupuytren's Contracture

The etiology of Dupuytren's contracture remains unclear (Fig. 15-1). Surgical treatment of Dupuytren's contracture remains the standard of care. The use of a transverse incision in the palm, which is then sutured, has been associated with the complication of hematoma formation. The advantages of leaving transverse wounds open are that a hematoma cannot form, and there is less pain and swelling in the hand, facilitating earlier finger motion. Histologically, myofibroblasts are the most important component in Dupuytren's disease. The fibroblastic proliferation in Dupuytren's contracture may be associated with an increase in platelet-derived growth factor B.

Acute Frostbite

In the past, the recommended management of acute frostbite of an extremity has varied. Currently, however, there is general agreement that rapid rewarming of the frozen extremity at a temperature of 40°C to 44°C is the most important component in the treatment of acute frostbite injury of an extremity. Frostbite of the hand in children may be severe enough to damage or destroy the growth plates in digits, which can result in significant bony deformities in adulthood.

Volkmann's Contracture

In chronic end-stage Volkmann's contracture in which a patient has no wrist or finger flexion and significant flexion contractures of the wrist and fingers with functioning wrist and finger extensors, the appropriate treatment should address a number of components of the impairment.

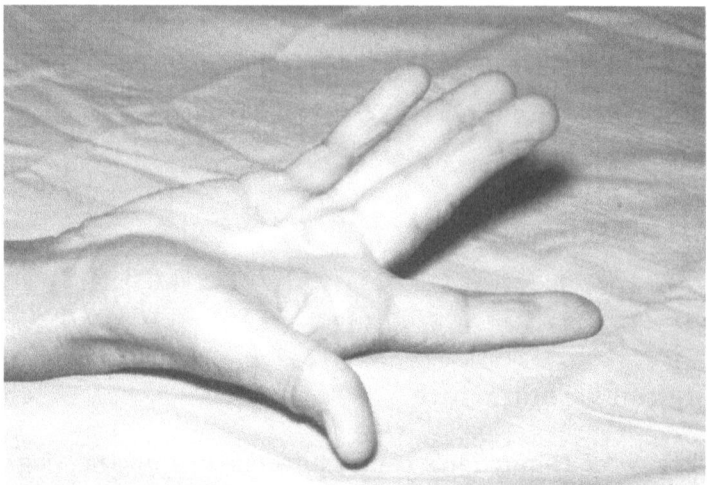

Fig. 15-1. A clinical photograph of a patient with Dupuytren's contracture involving the long, ring, and little fingers. The pretendinous cord can be seen in the palm involving that portion of the palmar aponeurosis and extending into the digital fascia, resulting in a flexion contracture of those digits.

Infarcted muscle should be excised in conjunction with tenotomies, for the purpose of regaining passive extension of the wrist and fingers. Neurolysis may be of some benefit. Tendon transfers can often restore wrist and finger flexion.

Burn Injury

Ankylosis and heterotopic bone formation of the elbow are recognized complications of burn injuries. Appropriate early treatment is active motion of the elbow. If ankylosis and heterotopic bone formation occur, surgical release of the joint and excision of the heterotopic bone are appropriate.

Reflex Sympathetic Dystrophy

Reflex sympathetic dystrophy is a complex clinical disorder that is ill-defined and poorly understood. Clinical findings of pain, atrophic changes, and vasomotor or anatomic dysfunction, with or without a previously recognized mechanical insult or trauma to the extremity, should raise suspicion of reflex sympathetic dystrophy. The diagnosis of reflex sympathetic dystrophy can best be confirmed using a sympathetic block. The most important features of successful treatment of RSD are early diagnosis, prompt initiation of physical therapy, and treatments that diminish sympathetic activity, such as a stellate ganglion block.

Suggested Reading

Amadio, P. C. 1988. Pain dysfunction syndromes. J. Bone Joint Surg. 70A:944.
Bigelow, D. R., and G. W. Ritchie. 1963. The effects of frostbite in childhood. J. Bone Joint Surg. 45B:122.
Green, D. P. 1993. Operative hand surgery, 3rd Ed., Chap. 13, 563.
Green, D. P. 1993. Operative hand surgery, Chap. 13, 2033.
Hand surgery update, 1994. The American Society for Surgery of the Hand, 26.1.
Hand surgery update. 1994. The American Society for Surgery of the Hand, 24–1.
McCash, C. R. 1968. The open palm technique in Dupuytren's contracture. Br. J. Plastic Surg. 17:271.
Terek, R. M., W. A. Jimaek, M. J. Goldberg, H. J. Wolfe, and B. A. Alman. 1995. The expression of platelet-derived growth factor gene in Dupuytren's contracture. J. Bone Joint Surg. 77A:1.

Questions

A. A 52-year-old man develops an ischemic contracture of the forearm as a complication of a cardiac catheterization. He presents to your clinic 6 months later. The hand is insensate, with severe flexion contractures of the wrist and fingers. He has significant pain in the forearm and hand and no active flexion of the wrist or fingers. His wrist and finger extensor function is intact. Recommended treatment should be:

1. Observation and follow-up examination
2. A wrist splint
3. Passive range of motion exercises and physical therapy, combined with dynamic splinting
4. Debridement of infarcted muscle, tenotomies, neurolysis, and tendon transfers
5. Amputation at the midforearm and a prosthesis

B. A 16-year-old girl is temporarily trapped in a car fire and sustains third-degree burns to her legs and no injury to her upper extremities. Six weeks later, she notices increasing loss of motion and pain in her right elbow. Initial radiographs had been unremarkable. Her right elbow motion was 40° to 130°.

Eight months later, she still has pain and her motion is now 75° to 95° in her right elbow. A lateral radiograph of the elbow is seen in Figure 15-2.

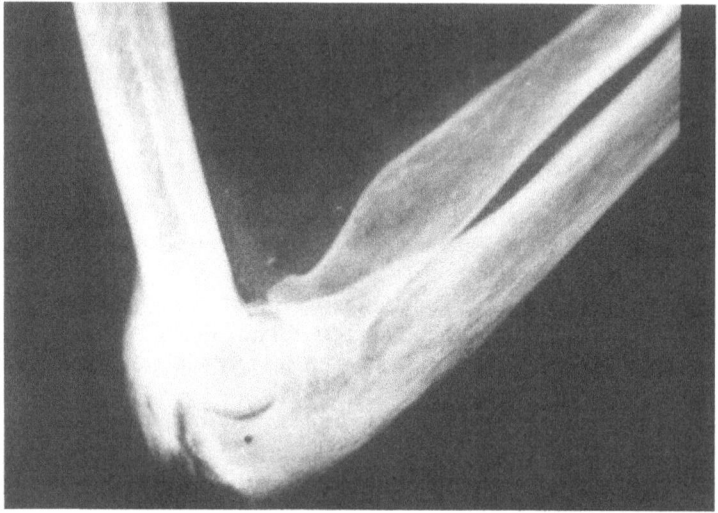

Fig. 15-2.

Recommended treatment should be:

1. Gentle active motion of the elbow
2. Active and passive motion of the elbow
3. Treatment with diphosphonates
4. Low-dose radiation treatment
5. Surgical excision/release of the elbow

C. A 57-year-old man has a palmar fasciectomy for treatment of Dupuytren's contracture. Closure of the wound is attempted with a Z-plasty technique; however, the transverse limbs cannot be closed. At this time, treatment should be:

1. Leave the palmar transverse wounds open
2. Cover the gaps with split-thickness skin grafts
3. Use a local transposition flap
4. Use a pedicle flap
5. Use a thenar flap

D. A 44-year-old astronaut is practicing for space walk maneuvers in his space suit in a vacuum chamber where temperatures are below $-170°C$. After 6 hours in the chamber, he exits complaining of bilateral hand pain. Examination shows that all of his digits are pale, white, and cold. Initial management should include:

1. Immersing both hands in a water bath that is between 22° and 25°C (room temperature)
2. Immersing both hands in a water bath that is between 37° and 38°C (core body temperature)
3. Immersing both hands in a water bath that is between 40° and 44°C
4. Giving the patient warm liquids and bandaging both hands in bulky dressings to allow rewarming at room temperature
5. Surgically debriding all tissues that do not show evidence of capillary refill, and administering antibiotics

E. The histology of Dupuytren's contracture appears related to the:

1. Myocyte
2. Myofibroblast
3. Fibroblast
4. Polymorphonuclear leukocyte
5. Chondrocyte

F. A 35-year-old female developed glossiness of the skin of her right hand, associated with some increased sweating, several months after a carpal tunnel release. She has progressively increasing discomfort in her hand and forearm, and the entire hand is hyperesthetic. This patient can best be treated with:

1. Elevation and night splinting
2. Physical therapy and cervical sympathetic blocks
3. Tranquilizers
4. Surgical release of Guyon's canal
5. Transcutaneous nerve stimulator

Answer Key

Chapter 1: Amputation and Replantation

A. 2
B. 5
C. 5
D. 4
E. 2

Chapter 2: Extensor Tendon Injuries

A. 4
B. 3
C. 5
D. 4

Chapter 3: Flexor Tendon Injuries

A. 3
B. 1
C. 4
D. 4
E. 4

Chapter 4: Soft Tissure Coverage

A. 4
B. 2
C. 5
D. 1

Chapter 5: Wrist Injuries

A. 5
B. 5
C. 3
D. 5
E. 3
F. 3
G. 4

Chapter 6: Tumors

A. 4
B. 3
C. 5
D. 4
E. 4
F. 5
G. 1
H. 2
I. 4

Chapter 7: Nerve Injuries (General Peripheral)

A. 4
B. 2
C. 4

Chapter 7: Nerve Injuries (Ulnar Nerve)

A. 5
B. 4
C. 4
D. 2

Chapter 7: Nerve Injuries (Radial Nerve)

A. 4
B. 2
C. 5
D. 1
E. 1

Chapter 7: Nerve Injuries (Median Nerve)

A. 5
B. 5
C. 2
D. 3
E. 1
F. 1
G. 5

Chapter 7: Nerve Injuries (Musculocutaneous Nerve)

A. 2

Chapter 8: The Thumb

A. 4
B. 5
C. 3

Chapter 9: Infections

A. 5
B. 5
C. 2
D. 4
E. 1
F. 1
G. 5
H. 3

Chapter 10: Arthritis

A. 1
B. 3
C. 2
D. 5
E. 4
F. 5
G. 3

Chapter 11: Tendon Transfers

A. 4
B. 2
C. 4
D. 2
E. 1
F. 2

Chapter 12: Brachial Plexus

A. 3
B. 3
C. 1
D. 4
E. 5
F. 1
G. 5

Chapter 13: Anatomy

A. 4
B. 4
C. 3
D. 4
E. 3
F. 3
G. 5
H. 3

Chapter 14: Congenital Anomalies

A. 3
B. 4
C. 5
D. 3
E. 3
F. 3

G. 5
H. 4
I. 5

Chapter 15: Miscellaneous

A. 4
B. 5
C. 1
D. 3
E. 2
F. 2

Index